Women Over Forty

Dr Anita Khokhar, M.D.
Professor
Dept. of Community Medicine
Vardhman Mahavir Medical College and Safdarjang Hospital
New Delhi

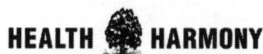

An imprint of
B. Jain Publishers (P) Ltd.
USA — Europe — India

WOMEN OVER FORTY

First Edition: 2012
1st Impression: 2012

All rights reserved. No part of this book may be reproduced, stored in a retrieval system or transmitted, in any form or by any means, mechanical, photocopying, recording or otherwise, without any prior written permission of the publisher.

© with the publisher

Published by Kuldeep Jain for

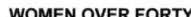
HEALTH HARMONY

An imprint of
B. JAIN PUBLISHERS (P) LTD.
1921/10, Chuna Mandi, Paharganj, New Delhi 110 055 (INDIA)
Tel.: +91-11-4567 1000 • *Fax:* +91-11-4567 1010
Email: info@bjain.com • *Website:* **www.bjain.com**

Printed in India by
J.J. Offset Printers

ISBN: 978-81-319-0869-3

भारत की राष्ट्रपति की चिकित्सक
राष्ट्रपति सचिवालय
राष्ट्रपति भवन
नई दिल्ली-110004
फोन: 011-23792985
फैक्स: 011-23793891
ई-मेल: parulbais@gmail.com

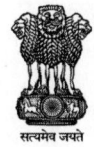

Physician to the President of India
President's Secretariat
Rashtrapati Bhavan
New Delhi - 11 0004
Tel. : 011-23792985
Fax: 011-23793891
E-mail: parulbais@gmail.com

FOREWORD

'Women Over Forty' written by Dr Anita Khokhar, M.D. is a synopsis of various ailments both physiological and pathological encountered by women. It gives a panoramic view of such conditions added by simplified illustrations and solutions to be easily understood by all. It will make an interesting reading for a non-medical person.

(Dr P.S. Bais)
Physician to the President

PREFACE

'I am not 40, I am 18 with 22 years of experience.'

-Unknown

Women have been playing multiple roles in their lives, be it that of a house wife, a working woman, a daughter, mother, wife, sister, aunt, grandmother or mother-in-law. In fact, someone once said, *'Women are fools trying to be everything to everyone.'* While carrying out their daily chores they often forget that they hold a key position in the family and society and life definitely revolves around them. They make this world whole and complete. Often we see them sacrifice their own needs and wants for those of others around her. Health is especially one vital issue which is put on the backburner. Women do not realise that if they themselves are not healthy, those around them will also be affected. As they grow older, not only do the demands and expectations from them increase but their chance of falling sick also increases. Women undergo a lot of transitions which affect their body and mind right from birth, menarche, childbirth to menopause. Over the years, longevity of women has increased which is further associated with an increase in the burden of middle age and old age related health problems. In fact, it was not until after 1900 that the average life expectancy of a woman actually exceeded the time at which most women would naturally encounter menopause. According to the independent projections of the United Nations Population Division, 95 per cent of future growth will occur in developing countries, with an increasing number and proportion of women aged 45 and over; their number will exceed 700 million before the turn of the century.

ACKNOWLEDGEMENTS

Apart from my efforts, the successful completion of this book depends largely on the encouragement and guidelines of many others. I take this opportunity to express my gratitude to the people who have been instrumental in the making of this book.

I would like to thank all those who provided astonishingly detailed and insightful comments, feedback and suggestions.

Especially,

1. Dr A. Sattar Yoosuf, Director, Department of Sustainable Development and Healthy Environments, WHO, SEARO, Delhi.
2. Dr SVS Deo, Professor, Surgical Oncology, IRCH, AIIMS.
3. Dr Sumit Sural, Professor, Department of Orthopedics, MAMC and LN Hospital, Delhi.
4. Dr Sanjay Pattnaiyak, Consultant Psychiatrist at VIHMHANS, Nehru Nagar, Delhi.
5. Dr Dinesh Mistry at north shore travel clinic Vancouver, Canada Area.

6. Dr Aparna Chawla, Psychiatrist registrar at Southern Health Melbourne Area, Australia
7. Dr Sharon Singsit, Registrar, Brimigham, UK.
8. Dr Parul Bais, Chief Physician to the honourable President of India, deserves a special thanks for going through the draft page by page and writing the foreword.

As with any such work, this book also rests on the prior work of others. Many archives, libraries and websites were accessed as a primary source for this book and I would like to acknowledge their input.

A lot of men have felt gender rivalry, if I may use the term, as they felt such books are required for men also. My previous book on Breast cancer and now this one both, focus on women's health, in particular. I promise to be unbiased next time.

A number of friends and acquaintances from across the globe via social networking sites ad e-mails have given their suggestions regarding the contents of the book and I thank them all.

A word of appreciation and gratitude is due to B Jain Publishers and the editing staff especially Ms. Somomita Taneja for her inputs in the book.

Finally, an honorable mention goes to my family and friends for their understanding and support.

PUBLISHER'S NOTE

With increasing modernization, women are becoming vulnerable towards the concept of ageing. The fortieth year of life signals the onset of a transition period from adulthood to old age. The lack of awareness to the issues approaching the life of a—women over 40—makes her behavior and approach towards life very imbalanced and chaotic.

The book give a total insight to the—anatomical, physiological, psychological and the social changes that a women over 40—faces. This is a time period when women should enjoy life—professionally and personally. This book serves as a guide to all those women who are combating with these problems; and also for those who are on the verge of coming to this age group. As we near forties we start to worry about ageing. Ageing is the sum total of all the changes that occur in our body with time. Growing old is a mixed bag. With age, though we gain experience and are better equipped to handle life, our body functions begin to decline. Several theories have been put forth to explain this complex process of ageing. An insight to all the issues creates a level awareness among this age group of women to deal with their life situations in a matured way so as to have solutions for all issues without much chaos and depression in life. This book is an attempt to overcome the issues of women over 40.

It gives me immense pleasure to present this book to the—women of today—so as to focus on the transition issues, which they may not be prepared to deal with, otherwise.

Kuldeep Jain
C.E.O., B. Jain Publisher's (P) Ltd.

CONTENTS

Foreword .... *iii*
Preface .... *v*
Acknowledgements .... *vii*
Publisher's Note .... *ix*

1. Anatomical and Physiological Changes 1
2. Female Reproductive System 15
3. Cervical Cancer 21
4. Breast Cancer 29
5. Ovarian Cancer 35
6. Cancer of the Uterus 43
7. Fibroids 49
8. Uterine Prolapse 57
9. Dysfunctional Uterine Bleeding 63
10. Menopause 65
11. Hormone Replacement Therapy (HRT) 79
12. Urinary Incontinence 89
13. Hypertension (High Blood Pressure) 97
14. Diabetes 111
15. Raised Cholesterol Level
    (Hypercholesterolaemia) 127

16.	Obesity	133
17.	Women and Heart Disease	141
18.	Osteoporosis	151
19.	Osteoarthritis	171
20.	Urinary Tract Infection (UTI)	177
21.	Thyroid Problems	183
22.	Mental and Psychological Problems	187
23.	Memory Loss	195
24.	Sexual Health	201
25.	Pregnancy After 40	207
26.	Contraception After 40	213
27.	Physical Fitness	221
28.	Diet	231
29.	Cosmetic Surgery	247
30.	Alternative Medicine	259
31.	Screening Tests for Women Over 40 Years	295
References		299

Chapter 1

Anatomical and Physiological Changes

Introduction

Reaching the fortieth year of life signals the onset of middle age. This age group is peculiar as it comes as a part of transition from adulthood towards old age. It usually lasts till 60 years of age. One is physically not at the prime of life and not old enough so that she retires from all her duties. At 40 today, women still have children to look after at home along with the professional front and may be a variety of other hobbies and interests in life. What leads to this gradual change from one phase to another is the process of ageing. If one is born, she has to age and it is an irreversible process no matter how much we try to reverse it. A lot of research has been done to find out what causes ageing and a few theories have been put forth too.

The theories of ageing have been grouped into two categories:

Programmed Theories

This theory introduces the concept of internal biological clock to explain the process of ageing from childhood. It has three subcategories.

1. As per the **endocrine theory,** production of some hormones like growth hormone and oestrogen decline with age.

2. As per the programmed **senescence theory,** T and the B lymphocytes under go programmed cell death.

3. As per the third theory that is, the **immunological theory,** with age, increased vulnerability to infections causes death.

Damage or Error Theories

This theory blames the external or environmental forces to gradually damage the internal cells and organs leading to ageing. It has six subcategories:

1. According to the first one, which is the **living theory,** ageing is the by-product of metabolism. That is, greater the organisms rate of metabolism, shorter is its life span and vice versa.

2. According to the second, all the damages within the body are caused by **oxygen free radicals** which cause ageing. An oxygen free radical is a by-product of normal metabolism produced when cells turn food and oxygen into energy. They damage proteins, membranes and nucleic acids, particularly DNA and organelles.

3. The accumulation of **cross linked proteins** damages cells and tissues besides slowing down bodily processes resulting in ageing.

4. As per the **wear and tear theory,** constant wear and tear of cells results, leading to damaged DNA. DNA damage leads to malfunctioning of genes, proteins, cells and deterioration of tissues and organs.

5. The fifth subcategory that is, **theory of error catastrophe** explains that damage to mechanisms that synthesise proteins, results in faulty proteins, which accumulate to a level that causes catastrophic damage to cells, tissues and organs.

6. Finally, as per the **somatic mutation theory,** genetic mutations occur and accumulate with increasing age, causing cells to malfunction.

Many of us feel sad or low about entering middle age but if one analyses the situation in detail, this is the time period when one could be enjoying life to the fullest as this is one of the most productive periods of a woman's life, both professionally and personally, that is, in her private life. One has a secure bank balance and can think of more than the career on one hand; on the other, too much of work takes its toll which could lead to a burnout and women decide to change to a lesser demanding job. Although many believe that their sex life suffers a setback during middle age, some women enjoy their sexual life more after menopause as they have no fear of becoming pregnant. Children have also grown up by now. Adolescent children are difficult to manage but they do not need constant supervision. However, thinking of their studies and future could be a cause of concern for many. Once one is well settled into marital life, the initial insecurities which are present in an arranged marriage disappear but life could be monotonous. If children leave the house or country for higher studies, it can lead to loneliness and depression as women experience what has been called the **'empty nest syndrome'.** Some could also be preparing to marry their children off. If the newly married couple comes and stays with the family, initially there could be a lot of stress because of maladjustment. And if three generations are staying together, there could be a problem of space as well. Becoming a grandparent brings a lot of joy to all. That is something most of the women look forward to. Increased health concerns of the self, spouse or older members of the family could be a constant source of tension. And God forbid, if the spouse dies, then there are more pressures to face. A large number of women join spiritual groups or religious organisations to help them overcome these difficulties.

As long as we realise that it is a part of a normal transitional phenomenon of life, one is better equipped to enter their fortieth year more confidently.

Anatomical and Physiological Changes in Women After the Age of 40

As we near forties we start to worry about ageing. Ageing is the sum total of all the changes that occur in our body with time. It refers not only to physical changes but also psychological and social changes that occur along with it. Growing old is a mixed bag. With age, though we gain experience and are better equipped to handle life, our body functions begin to decline. Many theories have been proposed to explain the process of ageing. The important ones have been listed. Several theories have been put forth to explain this complex process of ageing.

Hair

Greying of hair is the first thing that comes to our mind as we age. Greying can start in the thirties itself. The pigment which is responsible for the black colour of hair is **melatonin**. As we age, the hair follicles produce less melatonin resulting in the hair becoming grey and eventually white. Hair also looses density and becomes sparse. In women, the hair becomes less dense all over and the scalp becomes visible. It is the hair of the scalp which turn grey first of all followed by hair of the chest and pubic area. Hair is actually made up of protein and has a life of about 5 years when it falls and is replaced by new hair and the cycle goes on. Colour of the hair and time of greying is usually genetically determined. Once greying starts then it is an irreversible process.

Nail Changes

The nails become dull and brittle with age. The colour may change to yellow and look opaque. Nails, especially toe nails, may become hard and thick. Ingrown toe nails may be more common. Sometimes, lengthwise ridges develop on the nails which are a result of ageing. Some become brittle and break. Nail changes can also occur because of nutritional deficiency and infections.

Skin

Wrinkles are every woman's nightmare as we age! Skin is an important organ of our body. It helps us feel sensations, controls body temperature and electrolyte balance, and also protects from the environment.

Although the skin has many layers, it can be generally divided into three main parts:

1. The outer part or **epidermis** contains skin cells, pigment and proteins.

2. The middle part or **dermis** contains blood vessels, nerves, hair follicles and oil glands. The dermis provides nutrients to the outer layer.

3. The third layer under the dermis is the **subcutaneous layer** which contains sweat glands, some hair follicles, blood vessels and fat. Each layer also contains connective tissue with collagen fibres to give support and elastin fibres to provide flexibility and strength.

With age, the outer skin layer (epidermis) thins even though the number of cell layers remain unchanged.

The number of pigment-containing cells (melanocytes) decreases, but the remaining melanocytes increase in size. Ageing skin thus appears thinner, paler and translucent. Changes in the connective tissues reduce the skin's strength and elasticity. Blood vessels of the dermis become more fragile, which in turn leads to easy bruising and bleeding under the skin. Sebaceous glands produce less oil as you age. This can make it harder to keep the skin moist, resulting in dryness and itchiness. Also, sweating decreases with age; as a result there are higher chances of developing a heat stroke.

Smoking, stress and anxiety change the texture and colour of skin.

As the subcutaneous layer of fat, which provides insulation and padding, thins, it increases the risk of skin injury and reduces your ability to maintain body temperature. Skin tags, pigmented areas and blemishes are more common in old age. Climate, exposures to industrial and household chemicals, indoor heating, clothing, allergies to plants, other allergies and many other common exposures can also cause skin changes.

After the age of 40, there is a drop in circulating oestrogen which affects the elasticity of our skin. As women age, there is a decrease in the epidermis turnover rate which accounts for the doubling of time it might take to heal a wound. With age, the cell cycle slows down and cells cannot be renewed quickly. This causes the skin to become leathery and dull and more prone to the etching of wrinkles.

Muscle tone may be lost, causing a flabby or droopy appearance. A double chin may appear in some people. In some, the nose lengthens slightly and may look more prominent.

Ears

Ears may grow coarse hair in some. Wax becomes drier and wax glands fewer in number. This drier wax can impact and block the ear canal leading to difficulty in hearing.

Eyes

The eyebrows and eyelashes become grey. The skin around the eyelids, at the outer canthi of the eye turns into a 'crow's feet' pattern. The eyelids become droopy.

Teeth

Decay of teeth is also more common because as you age, the mouth becomes drier due to reduced secretion of saliva. The fillings start to chip and crack.

Loss of teeth can change the appearance of the face and also make chewing of food difficult. The jaw bone loses bone material, reducing the size of the lower face. Gums may also recede, contributing to dental problems and changes in the appearance of the mouth.

Vision Changes

With age, the lens inside the eye hardens and looses, its ability to focus. As a result, near vision gets affected. Initially one can hold the reading material a little farther away than usual but later more frequent changes in glasses occur. This is normal for age and is known as presbyopia.

Presbyopia worsens as you age and you will need vision correction at some point. However, this does not signify a disease process. With ageing there can be irritation and itching in the eye due to dryness. Your chances of macular degeneration, glaucoma and diabetic retinopathy also increase after the age of 40 which could lead to blindness if not checked in time. Peripheral vision decreases, ability to appreciate colour becomes less and later there could be an onset of cataract.

Hearing

Your ears have two jobs. One is hearing and the other is maintaining balance. Hearing occurs after vibrations cross the eardrum to the inner ear. They are changed into nerve impulses and carried to the brain by the auditory nerve.

Balance (equilibrium) is controlled in a portion of the inner ear. Fluid and small hair in the semicircular canal (labyrinth) stimulate the nerves that help the brain maintain balance.

As you age, your ear structures deteriorate. The eardrum often thickens and the bones of the middle ear and other structures are affected. It often becomes increasingly difficult to maintain balance.

Hearing may decline slightly with age. This age-related hearing loss is called presbycusis. Impacted ear wax is another cause of this trouble in hearing and it is more common with increasing age. In addition, the brain may have a slightly decreased ability to process or translate sounds into meaningful information.

Persistent, abnormal ear noise (tinnitus) is another fairly common hearing problem, especially for older adults. It is usually a result of mild hearing loss.

Taste and Smell

The senses of taste and smell interact closely, helping you appreciate food. Most taste really comes from odours. The sense of smell begins at nerve receptors, high in the membranes of the nose.

You have approximately 9,000 taste buds. Your taste buds are primarily responsible for sensing sweet, salty, sour and bitter tastes.

The number of taste buds decrease between the ages of 40 to 50 in women. Each remaining taste bud also begins to lose mass. If taste sensation is lost, usually salty and sweet tastes are lost first, with bitter and sour tastes lasting slightly longer.

Gastrointestinal Tract

In your forties, your bowel may begin to show wear and tear. You are more likely to develop lactose intolerance and be unable to consume milk products without subsequent gas, bloating and diarrhoea. Intestinal muscles lose their synchronous rhythm and as a result irritable bowel syndrome may develop which presents as diarrhoea, constipation, or both. More deposition of fat can also be associated with higher instances of gall stones.

Sleep

Efficiency of sleep also falls with age. With ageing one tends to sleep earlier and wake up earlier in the morning, or there is difficulty in falling asleep or these are frequent breaks in the sleep. The sleep cycle has two components –REM (rapid eye movements) sleep and NREM (non-rapid eye movements) sleep. By 35 years, the duration of stage 4 NREM sleep is only around 6 per cent of the total sleep time which is only half of what it is at 20 years. Wakefulness at night is prolonged and the duration of stage 1 NREM sleep is increased slightly by around 5 per cent of the total sleep time.

The percentage of REM sleep remains constant at around 22–25 per cent throughout early and middle adult life, but REM density gradually falls. Those in their forties find it difficult to adapt to changes in sleep pattern with change in environment and shift in work. During old age, although the sleep time at night is reduced, the day time naps are frequent. Thus, the total amount of sleep will be maintained. As the exposure to light falls in the elderly due to eye problems, or sickness, their sleep pattern gets influenced. Light exposure at night, even if it is brief, may reduce melatonin secretion and lead to insomnia. If one has an associated health condition or is on some medication, insomnia might be more common in them.

The main function of muscles is to carry out movement of the body. Contraction of the muscles helps in the return of venous blood to the heart. They also help in generating heat and hence maintaining body temperature. Muscles support the body; if they become weak there are chances a person will become more prone to falls and fractures.

As our age advances from 30, skeletal muscles atrophy and decrease in mass. As a result, the strength of muscles falls. The prominent loss of muscle tissue, usually seen in later years is commonly referred to as senile sarcopenia. With age, the number of muscle fibres, along with their size decreases. Also, non-contractile muscle fibres replace the active form. Accumulation of fat occurs as the lean muscle mass reduces. Less energy is released during metabolism by the mitochondria present within the muscles. So if energy intake does not decrease, one is likely to put on weight. Blood flow to the muscles reduces and so the motor neurons. Similarly, atrophy of the intercostal muscles leads to the development of deep depressions in between the ribs.

Bone density begins to decrease during the middle years of life. It is especially more so in women after they reach menopause. Reduction in the level of oestrogen, growth hormone along with reduced calcium and vitamin D absorption are mainly responsible for these changes. If the physical activity decreases, as is the usual norm in old age, there will be more bone loss as bone forming cells deposit calcium efficiently when a person undertakes weight bearing exercises. The loss of calcium from the aged skeleton commonly leads to the bones taking on the porous, sponge-like appearance. Vertebra and spine may become deformed leading to stooping. As the bones become too thin due to decalcification, there is a higher chance of fracture of the neck of the femur in older women as it is no longer able to support the weight of the body. The spinal column becomes curved due to thinning of vertebrae. Bone spurs, caused by ageing and overall use of the spine, may also form on the vertebrae.

The arches of the foot become less pronounced, contributing (slightly) to loss in height. The long bones of the arms and legs become more brittle because of mineral losses, but no change in length occurs and hence appear longer then the shortened torso.

Joints

As we age, the joint movement becomes stiffer and less flexible because the amount of lubricating fluid inside the joints decreases and the cartilage becomes thinner. Ligaments also tend to shorten and lose some flexibility, making joints feel stiff. Activity of the cartilage-forming cells (chondrocytes) decreases. As a result, there is reduction in the cartilage present in a joint. Such joints do not absorb shock well and are more susceptible to mechanical damage. Also, as bone to bone contact increases, joint pains become more common.

The outer portion of a joint capsule is composed of elastic ligaments, which bind the joint together, preventing dislocation while allowing free movement. With age, the elasticity of the collagen and elastin components of ligaments reduce resulting in reduced joint mobility, especially the ankle joint in women.

Hip and knee joints may begin to lose structure (degenerative changes). The finger joints lose cartilage and the bones thicken slightly. Finger joint changes are more common in women and may be hereditary. Common musculoskeletal problems like osteoarthritis, osteomalacia, osteoporosis, or muscle weakness sets in.

Heart

Heart muscle cells degenerate slightly with age. Ageing pigment—lipofiscin gets deposited and the valves become thicker and stiffer. In the elderly ladies, finding a murmur in the chest may be a normal finding. The heart rate may also slow as we age due to fibrous and fatty deposits in the sino atrial (SA) node, which is the natural pacemaker of the heart. The heart muscle wall thickens, so the amount of blood that the chamber can hold may actually decrease despite the increased overall size of the heart. Also, filling of the heart becomes slower.

Blood Vessels

Changes in the connective tissue of the blood vessels leads to their thickening. As a result, they become less flexible and thicker. This makes the heart work harder and hence, there is an onset of hypertension.

Bar receptors are the receptors which monitor blood pressure and make changes to maintain a constant blood pressure when a person changes positions or activities. These receptors become less sensitive with age. Therefore, as we age there are higher chances of experiencing dizziness or a sudden fall in blood pressure as we rise from lying position to standing, or from sitting to standing position.

Blood

Ageing causes a slight reduction in total body water which is normal. This results in decreased blood volume. The number of red blood cells are reduced which leads to fatigue. Lymphocytes, a type of white blood cells reduce resulting in a decreased ability to fight infection and resist it.

Brain

We become wiser as we age but there are certain other changes which are not so positive.

Changes in the brain occur with age but they are more pronounced in women in their sixties or seventies; brain begins to shrink. Areas like frontal lobe and hippocampus shrink more than the others. These areas play a role in mental ability and formation of new memories respectively.

The outer surface of the brain also begins to shrink. As the white matter decreases, cognitive functions like memory, attention, decision-making also become slow.

Chapter 2

Female Reproductive System

The female reproductive system comprises of the vagina, cervix, uterus, uterine (fallopian) tubes and ovaries.

Reproduction

In the reproductive process, two kinds of sex cells are involved. The male sperm and the female egg or ovum. These two cells meet in the female's reproductive system; the egg is fertilised in the uterine tube and implanted in the uterus. With age, the numbers of eggs are depleted, as a result women are no longer able to conceive.

Vagina

The vagina is a muscular, hollow tube that extends from the vaginal opening to the cervix of the uterus. It is situated between the urinary bladder and the rectum. Purposes of the vagina is to receive a male's erect penis and semen during sexual intercourse. It is also the exit canal for the bloody discharge during menstruation and the baby during a vaginal birth. It may also hold forms of birth control, such as a diaphragm, intrauterine device or a female condom. After menopause, due to a decrease in the amount of oestrogen, the vagina becomes dry causing itching and difficulty during sexual intercourse (dyspareunia). Post-menopausal changes of the vagina include loss of thick keratinised mucosa, decrease in the amount of glycogen produced by the vaginal epithelium and a decrease of fascial thickness underlying the mucosa. These changes are seen clinically as a thinning of the vaginal walls, loss of rugae and atrophy of vaginal size.

Cervix

The cervix is situated between the vagina and the uterus. Its mucous membrane helps to either allow for the passage of sperms or the obstruction of sperms. The sperm must pass through the cervix to reach an unfertilised egg. When a baby is born, it must pass through the cervix as it exits the uterus and enters the vagina. Cervical cancer is the greatest cancer concern for women. Annual pap smear cultures can monitor and detect abnormalities. Cervical cancer occurs most often in women over the age of 40.

Uterus

This muscular organ is made up of three layers, from deep to superficial—endometrium, myometrium and perimetrium. A fertilised egg implants itself into the wall of the endometrium where it will develop throughout the pregnancy. Post-menopausal changes of the uterus include a decrease in the size of the fundus relative to the cervix, a decrease in myometrial thickness and a thinning of the endometrium. Hormone replacement therapy will maintain some of the endometrial thickness but the size of the uterine fundus will decrease.

Fallopian Tubes or Uterine Tubes

The fallopian tubes extend off the uterus and connect with the ovaries. These tubes have finger-like projections called fimbrae at the end of the tube, near the ovary. These finger-like projections help to collect mature eggs released by the ovaries. Fertilisation of the egg happens mostly in the first one third of the fallopian tube.

Ovaries

Women have an ovary on each side of the uterus. Each month the ovaries release an egg which is then fertilised or sloughed off. They also produce oestrogen and progesterone which help with reproductive function.

The ovaries generally alternately release an egg every month. When an ovary ovulates or releases an egg, it is swept into the lumen of the uterine tube by the frimbriae. The post-menopausal ovary decreases in size even during use of hormone replacement. Any enlargement of the ovary should be considered a malignancy until proven otherwise.

Ageing Changes

Menopause is a normal part of a woman's ageing process. The ovaries stop releasing eggs (ova) and the menstrual periods stop. Most women experience menopause around the age of 50, although it occurs before the age of 40 in about 8 per cent of women. Prior to menopause, menstrual cycles often become irregular.

The ovaries become less responsive to stimulation by follicle stimulating hormone (FSH) and luteinizing hormone (LH). To try to compensate for the decreased response, the body produces more of these ovary stimulating hormones for a time. The level of these hormones will eventually decrease.

The hormones produced by the ovaries include the different forms of oestrogen (including oestradiol), progesterone and androgens (including testosterone). These hormones also decrease around menopause. The ovaries continue to produce small amounts of testosterone and some oestrogen. The hormones produced by the pituitary gland are also decreased.

Because hormone levels fall, changes occur in the entire reproductive system. The vaginal walls become less elastic, thinner and less rigid. The vagina becomes shorter. Secretions become scant and watery. The external genital tissue decreases and thins (atrophy of the labia).

In both men and women, reproductive system changes are closely related to changes in the urinary system.

Breast

Mammary glands, which are a part of the breasts, are very highly modified (sweat) glands. With age, a woman's breasts loses tissue and subcutaneous fat, reducing the size and fullness of the breast. There is also a decrease in the number of mammary glands, which the body replaces with fat tissue. These changes make the breasts less firm. The breasts also lose support.

Ageing breasts commonly flatten and sag and the nipple may turn in slightly. The area surrounding the nipple (the areola) becomes smaller.

Metabolism

Metabolism is at its peak when you are young and then with age it starts to become sluggish. One feels less inclined to undertake physical activity with age and also the loss of muscle mass contributes to this slow metabolism. If you are physically active then even at rest your muscles will burn more calories.

Female Reproductive System

In the forties, the thyroid gland's immunity producing related activities begin to wane. As a result, many of us develop hypothyroidism which could further lead to weight gain and the vicious cycle starts. More weight gain leads to work overload for pancreas which produces more insulin and as a result, more fatty substances are produced.

AGE TIME LINE	What happens to your skin as you get older?	30 More fine lines develop as collagen and elastin start to break down, and our delicate skin under the eyes begins to thin	45 + The skin become thinner, party because of hormonal changes, and more sensitive to irritative environmental factor and allergens. The skin losses much of its strength and elasticity
	25 Visible ageing of the skin starts and the skin replaces old cells more slowly	40 Deeper lines begin to etch around the mouth and eys. Forrows appear on the forehead and circles under the eyes.	50 + Age spots start to appear a common occurrence in more than 90 percent of fair-skinned people

There are two major components of facial ageing:

Dynamic lines
Muscular hyperactivity

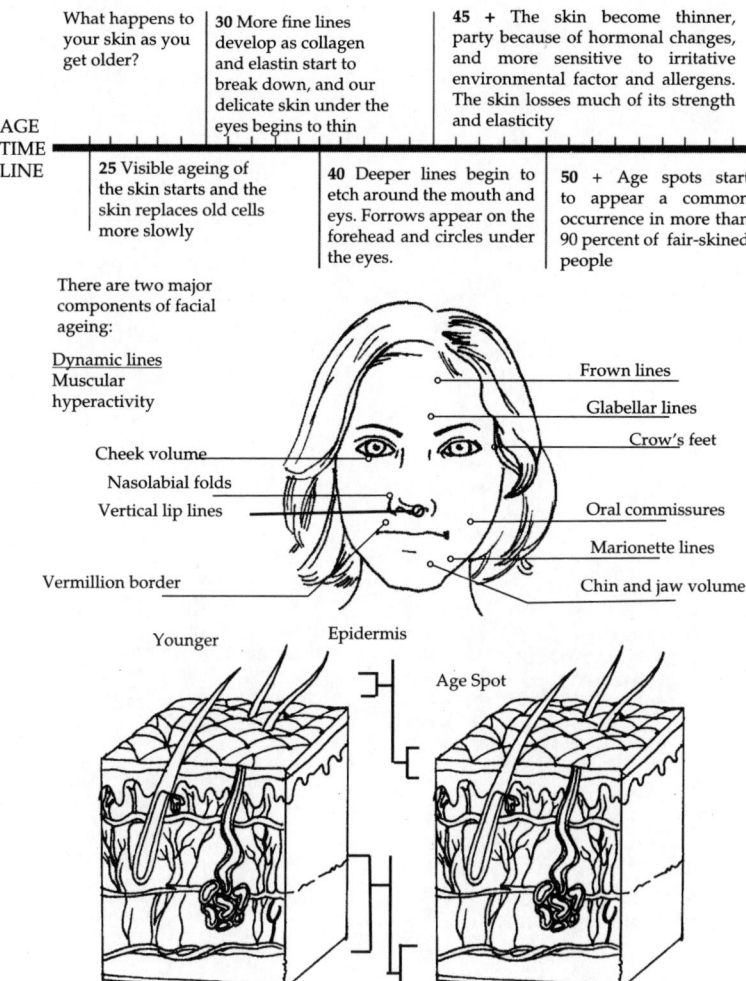

Fig 2.1: Subcutaneous fat layer

Chapter 3

Cervical Cancer

Cancer of the cervix is the second most common cancer to affect women. Even through this cancer is preventable, nearly 5 lakh cases are diagnosed with it every year; and nearly 3 lakh women die globally due to this cancer. Early detection of the disease can be effectively performed by screening but it is absent in areas where it is required the most, that is, in the developing countries. There are over 1 lakh new cases of cervical cancer occurring in India each year and it is responsible for 20 per cent of all the deaths of women. Keeping the countries with poor resources in mind, WHO recommends that at least one screening should be done for women between the age of 35 to 40 years. It has been seen that over 80 per cent women with invasive cervical cancer have not had a pap test in the past 5 years.

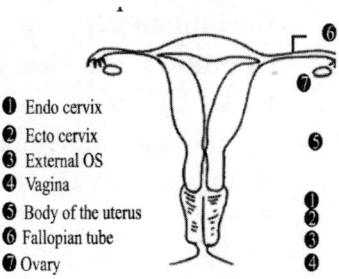

❶ Endo cervix
❷ Ecto cervix
❸ External OS
❹ Vagina
❺ Body of the uterus
❻ Fallopian tube
❼ Ovary

Fig. 3.1: Anatomy of the uterus and cervix

Cervix

Cervix is the lower part of the womb which forms a canal that leads outside the body of the female.

Cancer of the Cervix

Cervical cancer is one disease which gives a warning of its occurrence in the future by means of a precancerous condition. In precancerous conditions, cells of the cervix appear abnormal but the cancer has yet not set in. It gives the first hint to the doctor for cervical cancer which will develop in later years. Since most of these conditions do not cause any symptoms, they are usually picked up by a pap test or a pelvic examination.

Once the abnormal cells spread deep into the cervix or to other tissues outside the cervix, diagnosis of cervical cancer is made. Although cervix is a part of the uterus, cancer of the cervix is different from cancer of the uterus and the management is also not the same.

High Risk Factors

The following have been suggested as risk factors for cervical cancer:

1. Sex without using condoms results in infection with the human papilloma virus (HPV).
2. Conditions which weaken the immunity of a person to fight a disease like HIV.
3. As the age increases so do the chances of suffering from cervical cancer. It is more common after 40 years of age.
4. Smoking.
5. Low socio-economic level which is commonly associated with poor genital hygiene, early marriage and multiple childbirths.

6. Having sexual intercourse before the age of 18.

7. Having multiple sexual partners.

Symptoms

In the initial stages, cervical cancer is without any symptoms. That is why screening with a pap test is of utmost relevance as it can pick up abnormal cells.

1. Abnormal vaginal bleeding other than the regular period, bleeding after sexual intercourse or a pelvic exam.

2. Heavier periods which last for more number of days.

3. Foul smelling discharge.

4. Low back pain.

5. Pain during urination.

6. Pain during sex (dyspareunia).

Once the cancer spreads to other organs, it may lead to constipation, passing of blood in the urine, or an abnormal opening in the cervix.

Diagnosis

1. **Pap Test:** It is a term most of us are familiar with. It is not only simple to perform but is also quick to perform without causing discomfort to the lady. It is recommended for the first time when a lady becomes sexually active and once a year thereafter. It is this test which allows us to look for any abnormal cells which could indicate either a premalignant condition or frank cancerous changes is the woman's cervix, under the microscope. None of the investigations are totally fool proof and the same applies to pap test as some (very few) women develop cervical cancer in spite of regular pap tests.

The best time for a pap test is between 10 and 20 days after the first day of her menstrual period, when the lady is not menstruating. For about two days before testing, a woman should avoid douching or using spermicidal foams, creams, jellies, or vaginal medicines (except as directed by the physician). These agents may wash away or hide any abnormal cervical cells.

The woman is asked to lie on her back. A speculum is then inserted into the birth canal to view the vagina and cervix from inside. Before that, the outside structures are also looked at carefully in case there is any change in them. A small brush called a cervical brush is then inserted into the opening of the cervix (the cervical os) and turned around to collect a sample of cells. Another sample is taken by scraping the area surrounding the cervical opening and not going inside it (See Fig. 3.2).

Both the samples are gently smeared on a glass slide, fixed and sent to a lab where the samples are analysed by a pathologist. The results of the pap smear are usually available within two to three weeks.

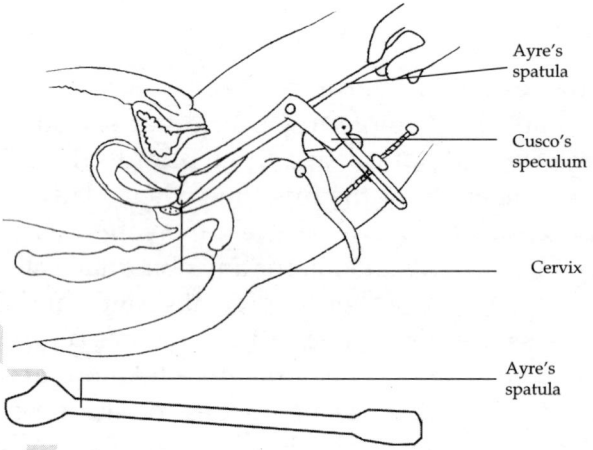

Fig. 3.2: Cusco's speculum and Ayre's spatula

2. **Pelvic Examination**: It is a part of routine examination for a woman. The doctor not only looks at the reproductive organs but also feels them with his gloved hand.

3. **Biopsy:** In this investigation, a piece of cervical tissue is removed and sent to a pathologist for examination. There are several types of cervical biopsies that may be used to diagnose cervical cancer. Some procedures require local anaesthesia, while others require general anaesthesia. These various types of biopsies include:

    i. *Loop Electrosurgical Excision Procedure (LEEP)*: A procedure which uses an electric wire loop to obtain a piece of tissue.

    ii. *Colposcopy*: Colposcope, an instrument with a magnifying lens is used to visualise the cervix. If abnormal tissue is found, a biopsy is usually performed (colposcopic biopsy).

    iii. *Endocervical Curettage (ECC)*: A procedure which uses a narrow instrument called a curette to scrape the lining present on the inner side of the cervical canal.

    iv. *Cone Biopsy (Conisation)*: A biopsy in which a larger cone-shaped piece of tissue is removed from the cervix by using the loop electrosurgical excision procedure.

    v. *Cold Knife Cone Biopsy*: A procedure in which a laser or a surgical scalpel is used to remove a piece of tissue.

4. Blood Tests.

5. **Radiological Investigations:** Like ultrasonography, CT scan and chest X-ray are also carried out which help in staging the disease and unless the staging of the disease is done, a definite treatment cannot start.

Treatment

Treatment may include:

1. Surgery

    Cryosurgery: Use of liquid nitrogen or a probe that is very cold, to freeze and kill cancer cells.

    Laser Surgery: Use of a powerful beam of light, which can be directed at specific parts of the body without making a large incision, to destroy abnormal cells.

    Hysterectomy: Surgery to remove the uterus, including the cervix. In some cases, a hysterectomy may be required, particularly if abnormal cells are found inside the opening of the cervix.

2. Radiation Therapy.
3. Chemotherapy.

LEEP or **Conisation** may also be used to remove abnormal tissue.

Prevention

The following protective factors may decrease the risk of cervical cancer:

1. Avoid being exposed to HPV infection by adhering to the following:

    i.   Not having sex at an early age.

    ii. Having safe, protected sex using condoms.

    iii. Not having many sexual partners.

    iv. Not having a partner who has had many sex partners.

2. Avoid smoking as it is a known carcinogen.

Get vaccinated: Vaccines have been developed that can protect women from HPV infections. So far, a vaccine that protects against HPV types 6, 11, 16 and 18 that is, Gardasil has been approved for use in this country by the FDA. It protects from the two most important HPV types which are responsible for more than 90 per cent of genital warts. A series of three injections are given over a 6 month period. The second injection is given 2 months after the first one and the third is given 4 months after the second. Side effects other than swelling and redness at the site of injection are rare. This vaccine only works to prevent HPV infection—it will not treat an infection that is already there. The ideal time of giving the vaccine is before a girl becomes sexually active. The American Cancer Society also recommends that the vaccine should be routinely given to females aged 11 to 12. Since the vaccine does not protect against all cancer-causing types of HPV, a routine screening with pap tests cannot be replaced. Pap tests are still necessary.

Chapter 4

Breast Cancer

Breast remains the leading area to be affected by cancer among women in the developed world. It is also the leading cause of death amongst them. In developing countries, due to adoption of a western lifestyle, the disease is increasing very fast in magnitude. As of now, we do not have enough knowledge about the cause of this dreaded disease. Hence, prevention of this disease is not practically possible. What is possible is early detection of the disease by screening of women for breast disease.

High Risk Factors

1. **Age:** The risk of breast cancer increases as the woman gets older. It is common after the age of 40 years although age is no bar.

2. **Early Menstruation and Late Menopause:** The influence of hormones that is, oestrogen and progesterone are involved in the onset of breast cancer.

3. **Late Marriage and Late Full Term Pregnancy:** An early full time pregnancy seems to have a protective effect. Women whose first pregnancy is delayed to their late thirties are at a higher risk than women who have borne many children.

4. **Genetic Predisposition:** The risk of suffering from breast cancer increases if any of the family members (mother, sister and daughter) have had breast cancer. The younger the family member at the time of developing the cancer, the greater the risk. Those with a family history of bilateral (involving both the breasts) cancers are at an increased risk. Having genetic mutation in the breast cancer genes BRCA1 or BRCA2 also increases the risk.

5. **Socio-economic Status:** It is more common in women from higher socio-economic groups because of an affluent lifestyle. Higher age at first childbirth and not breast feeding the child also increases the risk.

6. **Radiation Therapy:** Women whose breasts are exposed to radiation under the age of 30 years are at a higher risk of developing cancer later in life.

7. **Diet, Alcohol and Smoking:** A diet high in fats, consumption of moderate amounts of alcohol and smoking increase the risk.

8. **Obesity:** Weight gain as an adult or weight gain after menopause creates an added risk. Higher levels of oestrogen production in obese women probably also has a role to play.

9. **Personal History of Breast Cancer:** Women who have had cancer in one breast have an increased risk of getting it in the other breast.

10. **Oral Contraceptives and Hormone Replacement Therapy (HRT):** Combined hormone replacement therapy in Women's Health Initiative Trial has shown the risk of breast cancer to increase.

11. **Race and Ethnicity:** White women have a higher incidence of breast cancer as compared to African-American women after the age of 40 years while African-American women have a higher incidence before the age of 40. In contrast, African-American women are more likely to die from breast cancer at all ages.

12. **Abnormal Breast Biopsy:** Some types of benign breast conditions are more closely linked to breast cancer risk than others.

Symptoms

1. Lump or mass in the breast / armpit.
2. Change in the shape and size of the breast.
3. Nipple discharge (especially blood).
4. Skin changes like dimpling, skin resembling that of an orange peel or retraction of the nipple.

Age (Years)	BSE	CBE	Mammogram
20	Monthly	Nil	Nil
20-39	Monthly	Every 3 Years	Nil
40 and over	Monthly	Yearly	Once a Year

Diagnosis

Breast self-examination should be performed on a regular basis by all women. A thorough clinical examination by your physician can reveal a lump at an early stage. Following are the investigations usually required to reach the final diagnosis:

Mammograms

An X-ray of the breast (mammogram) is the best tool available for early diagnosis even before symptoms appear. X-ray is taken after placing the breast in direct contact with an ultra-sensitive film. Mammograms can often detect a breast lump and can also show small deposits of calcium in the breast. Although most calcium deposits are benign, a cluster of very tiny specks of calcium (called microcalcifications) may be an early sign of cancer. In young women in whom breasts are denser and more fibrous, a small percentage of breast cancers may not be visible on a mammogram, which otherwise may or may not be palpable by BSE (Breast self examination) or CBE (Clinical breast examination).

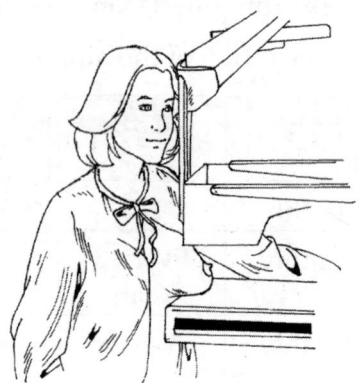

Fig. 4.1: Mammography

Ultrasonography

Using high frequency sound waves, ultrasonography can often show whether a lump is a fluid filled cyst (not cancer) or a solid mass (which may or may not be cancer). It is particularly useful in young women with dense breasts in whom mammograms are difficult to interpret. It can also be used to localise impalpable breast lumps.

Fine Needle Aspiration Cytology (FNAC)

A thin needle is put into the lump/mass and a tiny amount of fluid and/or cells are removed from the breast lump and then smeared on to a slide to be checked by a pathologist. It is the least invasive technique of obtaining cells for diagnosis. False negatives do occur and invasive cancer cannot be distinguished from in situ disease. Ultrasound guided FNAC is a better technique, as it is more likely to get cells from the lump.

Needle Biopsy

Using a fine needle such Trucut or Corecut biopsy device under local anaesthesia tissue can be removed from the lump or an area that looks suspicious on the mammogram but cannot be felt. Tissue removed in a needle biopsy goes to a lab to be checked by a pathologist for cancer cells. Invasive cancer can be distinguished from in situ disease with needle biopsy.

Surgical Biopsy

In an incision biopsy, the surgeon cuts out a portion of a lump or suspicious area. In an excision biopsy, the surgeon removes the entire lump or suspicious area and an area of healthy tissue around the edge of the lump. A pathologist then examines the tissue under a microscope to check for cancer cells. A biopsy should not be performed before mammography as it may interfere with the interpretation of the results.

Treatment

Depends on the type of breast cancer. However, basic modalities remain the same that is, chemotherapy, surgery, radiation therapy and immunotherapy.

Outcome

The best indicators of the likely course of the disease and its outcome in breast cancer are the tumour size and lymph node involvement. Prognosis depends not on the duration for which the tumour has been present but on its invasiveness and metastatic potential. In an attempt to define which tumour will behave aggressively and require early systematic treatment, a host of prognostic factors have been described like hormone receptor status, histological grading of tumour, oncogene and growth factor analysis.

Chapter 5

Ovarian Cancer

The ovaries are more easily understood as an egg sac in a woman's body. Ovaries produce eggs and the female hormones – oestrogen and progesterone, which further control development of the female body characteristics, menstruation and pregnancy. There are two ovaries, one on either side of the uterus (See Fig. 5.1).

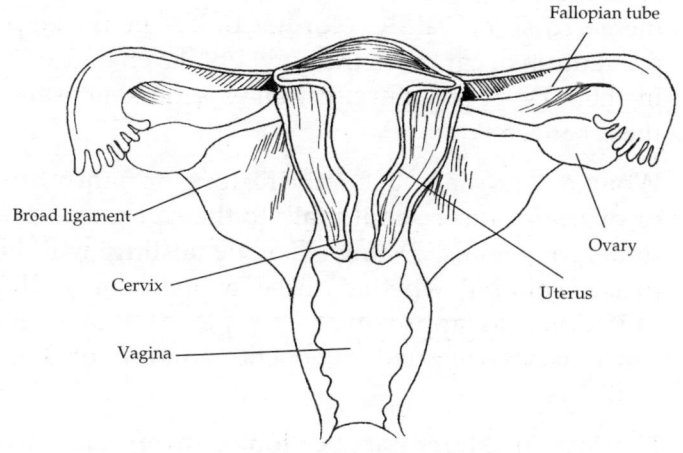

Fig. 5.1: Reproductive system

Ovarian cancer ranks at number eight amongst women cancers and is the fifth leading cause of cancer deaths in women.

High Risk Factors

1. **Age:** The risk of ovarian cancer increases with age and most are diagnosed only after they have reached menopause. According to the National Cancer Institute, the highest incidence of ovarian cancer occurs in women over the age of 60 years.

2. **Family History of Ovarian Cancer:** Having a family history of breast cancer amongst close relatives like mother or sisters increases the risk of developing this disease. For those with such a history the risk is 5 per cent more as against 1.5 per cent for those with no family history of ovarian cancer.

3. **Genetics:** BRCA1 (breast cancer gene 1) and BRCA1 (breast cancer gene 2) are two genes responsible for breast cancer. If they undergo any mutation, the risk of developing both, breast cancer and ovarian cancer increases significantly. Normal BRCA genes help in prevention of cancer in the body but if a change occurs in their DNA structure, it makes a person prone to these cancers.

   Women who have a family history of either breast or ovarian cancer should talk to their physicians and undergo genetic testing. Genetic testing will help in determining whether these women carry BRCA mutations, as approximately 9 per cent of ovarian cancer cases are due to a genetic mutation of BRCA1 or BRCA2.

4. **History of Hereditary Colon Cancer:** Hereditary cancer of the colon is a condition which develops in

the younger population, usually less than 40 years of age and is due to the inherited genes. Along with colon cancer, it also increases the chances of ovarian and endometrial cancer in women.

5. **Early Menstruation/Late Menopause:** Women who begin menstruating before the age of 12 years or those who do not reach menopause until after the age of 50 years, are at an increased risk for ovarian cancer as well as breast cancer. This may be because women who have more menstrual cycles throughout their lifetime are at a higher risk of ovarian and breast cancer. Research suggests that women who become pregnant, breast feed, or take birth control pills are at a lower risk of developing ovarian cancer.

6. **Personal/Family History of Breast Cancer:** Women who have been diagnosed with breast cancer have an increased risk of developing ovarian cancer because many of the risk factors for breast cancer (including early menstruation, late menopause, delayed childbirth and BRCA gene mutations) also put the woman at the risk for ovarian cancer.

7. **Medications:** Having taken fertility drugs or hormone therapy after menopause may increase the chances of ovarian cancer. Oral contraceptive pills, although hormonal in nature slightly decrease the chances of developing ovarian cancer.

8. **Obesity:** Deaths from ovarian cancer are higher among obese women as compared to normal weight women.

9. **Talcum Powder Use:** Women who regularly apply talcum powder to their genitals are at a slightly increased risk of developing ovarian cancer.

Symptoms

Although symptoms with which a woman presents with ovarian cancer may differ from one person to another, the following are the most common symptoms:

1. Sensation of pressure or pain in the abdomen or pelvis.
2. Persistent, gas, nausea and indigestion.
3. Frequency of passing urine is increased in the absence of an infection.
4. Unexplained changes in bowel habits.
5. Unintentional weight gain or weight loss, particularly weight gain in the abdominal region.
6. Pain during intercourse.
7. Feeling of tiredness and fatigue.
8. Leg pain.
9. Ovarian cancer usually gets diagnosed at a later stage because it does not produce any symptoms earlier on and whatever symptoms that the patient experiences are often vague and non-specific.

Diagnosis

First the medical history is taken and then a general examination is performed followed by pelvic a examination. The following tests may be asked for to reach a diagnosis:

1. **Ultrasound:** Of the abdomen to look at major organs like the uterus, kidneys and liver.
2. **Computed Tomography (CT or CAT scan):** The CT scan may indicate enlarged lymph nodes—a possible sign of a spreading cancer beyond ovaries.

3. **Lower Gastrointestinal (GI) Series:** X-rays of the colon and rectum using a contrast dye called barium.

4. **Intravenous Pyelogram (IVP):** Special X-ray of the kidneys and ureters after injecting a dye.

5. **Blood Test:** Is used to measure a substance in the blood called CA-125 which is a tumour marker. It may be elevated in conditions other than ovarian cancer also. The presence of tumour marker helps in monitoring the progress of treatment for ovarian cancer.

6. Biopsy.

Role of Prophylactic Oophorectomy

Prophylactic oophorectomy means removal of ovaries in high risk women so that actual cancer of ovaries does not occur.

A physician will help you assess your risk of ovarian cancer based on the following:

1. A personal history of breast cancer diagnosed before menopause.

2. A known mutation of the breast cancer genes—BRCA1 or BRCA2, in your family.

3. A first degree relative, such as your mother, sister or daughter, with onset of breast cancer or ovarian cancer before the age of 50 years.

4. A family history of ovarian cancer in two or more relatives.

5. A male family member with breast cancer.

After having determined the individual risk of a person for ovarian cancer, a genetic counsellor discusses the pros and cons of prophylactic oopherectomy.

Treatment

1. **Surgery:** Ovaries may be removed and the surgical procedure is known as oophorectomy. Also depending on the spread of the cancer, fallopian tubes and uterus may also be removed. For ovarian cancer patients, an omentectomy is usually combined with the removal of ovaries and uterus. In this procedure, a fold of abdominal tissue is also removed.

    Debulking is done to remove as much of the tumour as possible. It can be done before starting chemotherapy, or radiation therapy, or in case the cancer has spread, to improve the outcome of the disease.

2. **Chemotherapy.**
3. **Radiation Therapy.**

Prevention

Although cancer of the ovaries cannot be prevented, certain tests can be done to spot it at the earliest:

1. **Pelvic Examination:** Annual internal examination starting at the age of 18 should be advocated. Physicians perform pelvic exams to check for abnormalities in the size or shape of the uterus, vagina, ovaries, fallopian tubes, bladder and rectum.

2. **Genetic Testing:** It is done to determine whether women carry mutations of the BRCA1(breast cancer gene 1) or BRCA1 (breast cancer gene 2) genes. The decision to undergo genetic testing should be made carefully with inputs from the physician and family members.

3. **Pregnancy and Breast Feeding:** If a woman becomes pregnant with her first child before the age of 30, it decreases the chances of ovarian as well as breast cancer. This is because there is an interruption of menstrual cycles during pregnancy. Women who never become pregnant are at a higher risk of ovarian cancer and breast cancer than those who have a child before the age of 30. The older a woman is, the more likely her ovarian and breast tissues have already been exposed to some cancer-causing substances called carcinogens. Therefore, exposure to elevated hormonal levels during pregnancy at a later age may stimulate the growth of abnormal ovarian or breast tissue. Likewise, breast feeding also decreases the risk of ovarian and breast cancer.

4. **Birth Control Pills:** Use of oral contraceptives seems to lower the risk for ovarian cancer. As per American Cancer Society, women who take birth control pills for at least 5 years decrease their chances of ovarian cancer by 60 per cent. The risk appears to be greater the longer a woman takes birth control pills.

5. **Tubal Ligation or Hysterectomy:** Procedures to tie the fallopian tubes or remove the uterus lower the risk of ovarian cancer. But these procedures should never be done just to decrease the chances of ovarian cancer as they are associated with certain complications of their own.

6. **Prohylactic Oophorectomy:** As a procedure, this is not commonly performed. Although removal of the ovaries will remove the main source of oestrogen from the body and decrease the chances of ovarian cancer. Your personal risk assessment, as mentioned before, is a must.

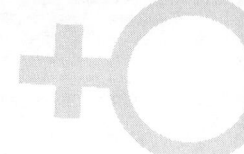

Chapter 6

Cancer of the Uterus

Womb or the uterus is a common site for gynaecological problems for women especially, during middle age.

Other than cancer of the cervix, which is also a part of the uterus, the rest of the tumours arising from various parts of the uterus (Fig. 6.1) are referred to as uterine cancer.

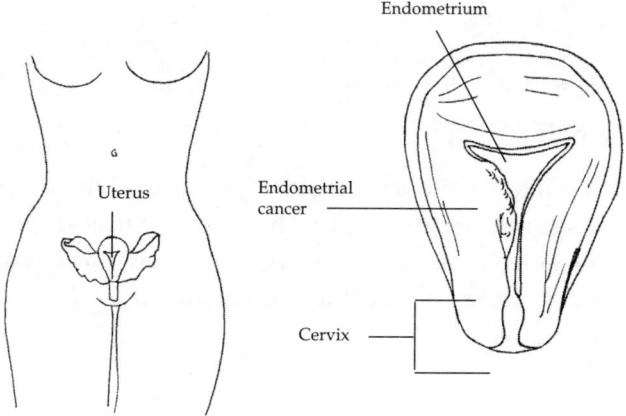

Fig. 6.1: Parts of the uterus

Risk Factors

Some of the known risk factors for uterine cancer are:

1. Age over 50 years.
2. History of endometrial hyperplasia.
3. Oestrogen replacement therapy.
4. Overweight and obesity.
5. Diabetes.
6. High blood pressure.
7. History of other cancers.
8. History of taking Tamoxifen for breast cancer treatment or prevention.

Symptoms

Unusual vaginal bleeding or discharge, especially after menopause.

Pain during urination.

Pain during sexual intercourse.

Pain in the pelvic area.

Any recurrence of vaginal bleeding around the time of menopause should be thoroughly checked and investigated. It should not be taken casually as a part of menopause as most of the cases of uterine cancer occur at the time menopause begins.

Diagnosis

To reach a diagnosis of uterine cancer, first of all a detailed history and physical examination is carried out. After that the following may be carried out:

1. **Pelvic Examination:** A thorough pelvic examination to check organs like vagina, ovaries, rectum, bladder, etc.

2. **Dilation and Curettage (D and C):** In this, a minor procedure is carried out where a curette is used to scrape the internal lining of the cervical canal and uterus.

3. **Transvaginal Ultrasound:** A probe is inserted via the vagina into the uterus to look at the thickness and texture of the inner layer of the uterus.

4. **Endometrial Biopsy:** Tissue from the uterine lining is removed so that the sample of cells from the uterine lining can be examined under the microscope. This procedure does not require general anaesthesia.

5. **Pap Test**.

To find out the extent of spread of cancer, the following tests may be required:

1. Blood tests.
2. Chest X-rays.
3. Computed tomography (CT or CAT) scans of various sections of the abdomen.
4. Ultrasound of the abdomen.
5. Special exams of the bladder, colon and rectum.

Treatment

1. **Surgery:** Surgery is the most common treatment for endometrial cancer. Removal of the uterus along with removal of the fallopian tubes and ovaries may be required depending upon the spread of cancer.

2. **Radiation:** Radiation therapy involves the use of high dose X-rays to kill cancer cells. It can be given from outside the body and from inside of the uterus (brachytherapy). Brachytherapy has fewer side effects than the external radiation therapy, but it treats only a small area of the body.

3. **Hormone Therapy:** Treatment with progestin may be an option for women with early endometrial cancer who want to have children at a later date and do not want their uterus to be removed because of this reason. The outcome of treatment should be carefully discussed with the patient as the cancer might return after this therapy. Gonadotropin releasing hormone agonists can also be prescribed as these drugs can lower oestrogen levels in premenopausal women.

4. **Chemotherapy:** Women with advanced stages of endometrial cancer that is, stage III and IV undergo treatment with chemotherapeutic drugs along with other modalities of treatment.

As is essential with the treatment of other cancers, follow up is advised to determine if the cancer returns.

Outcome

Because endometrial cancer is usually diagnosed in the early stages (70 per cent to 75 per cent of cases are in stage I at the time of diagnosis; 10 per cent to 15 per cent of cases are in stage II; 10 per cent to 15 per cent of cases are in stage

III or IV), there is a better progress in or outcome associated with it than with other types of gynaecological cancers such as cervical or ovarian cancer. About 75 per cent to 95 per cent of stage I patients survive for 5 years.

Prevention

The following can reduce the chances of endometrial cancer:

1. **Hormone Therapy (HT):** Replacing oestrogen alone after menopause may increase your risk of endometrial cancer. Taking synthetic progestin, a form of the hormone progesterone, with oestrogen causes the lining of the uterus to shed. This kind of combination hormone therapy lowers your risk of uterine cancer but hormone therapy is associated with its own side effects (details mentioned in chapter on HRT).

2. **Oral Contraceptives:** Use of oral contraceptives can reduce endometrial cancer risk, even 10 years after you stop taking them.

3. **Maintaining a Healthy Weight:** Obesity is one of the most significant risk factors for the development of endometrial cancer. You can help prevent endometrial cancer by maintaining a healthy weight. Excessive fat tissue can increase levels of oestrogen in your body, which increases your risk of endometrial cancer and breast cancer. Maintaining a healthy weight as you age, lowers your risk of endometrial cancer as well as other diseases.

4. **Exercise:** Regular exercise can cut down the risk of endometrial cancer. Women who exercise daily have half the risk of endometrial cancer compared with women who do not exercise, according to the American Cancer Society.

Chapter 7

Fibroids

Fibroids are growths made of muscle and connective tissue that originate from the wall of the uterus. Uterine fibroids are among the most common tumours in women. The process of formation of a fibroid is the same as the formation of any other growth in the body, that is, single cells multiply to produce a growth which is commonly described as pale, firm and rubbery. This growth or mass is distinct from the nearby tissues. Any such growth which develops in the body is called a tumour, but fibroids are not cancerous. Fibroids develop in the period between puberty and menopause indicating that female reproductive hormones play a role in fueling their growth. Fibroids are very common. They occur most often in women between the ages of 30 and 50, although women in their twenties sometimes have them.

It is not uncommon to have more than one fibroid. They are usually round to oval in shape with variable sizes. They are named according to the part of the uterus where they are found. Fibroids that grow inside the wall of the uterus are called **intramural fibroids**. Fibroids that grow outward from the wall of the uterus into the abdominal cavity are called **subserosal fibroids**. Fibroids that grow inward from the uterine wall, taking up space within the cavity of the uterus, are called **submucosal fibroids**. A fibroid that is attached to the uterus by a thin stalk is called a **pedunculated fibroid**. If you have a fibroid, knowing these terms will give a better understanding of the fibroid (See Fig. 7.1).

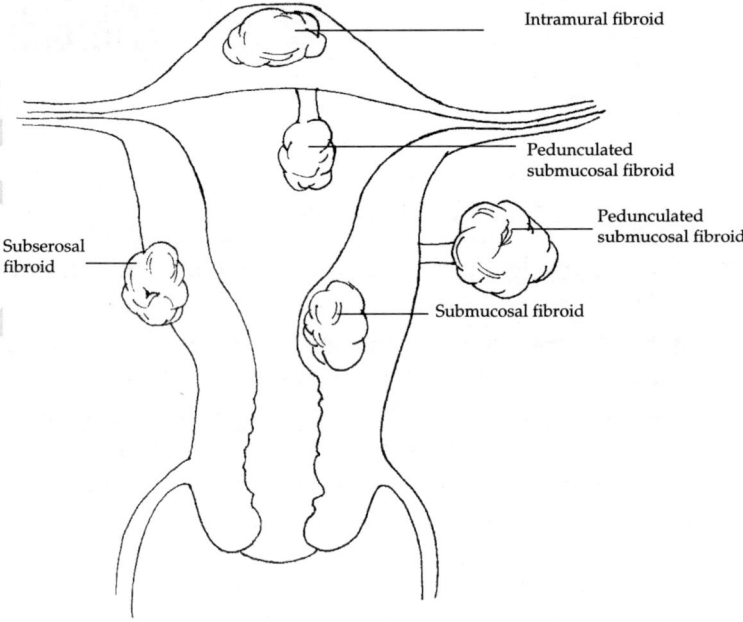

Fig. 7.1: Types of fibroids of the uterus

Symptoms

Most of the fibroids manifest no signs and symptoms and hence, women are unaware of their presence. Many are found incidentally by the doctor during a pelvic examination or an ultrasound procedure. Fibroids cause problems for about 1 in 4 women, most frequently during their thirties or forties.

The most common symptoms include:

1. Heavy bleeding at the time of menstrual period.
2. Periods lasting for more number of days or bleeding in between periods.
3. Discomfort, or pressure, or pain which is felt in the pelvic area.
4. Urinary incontinence, frequent urination, or not being able to pass the entire quantity of urine, some is retained in the bladder.
5. Constipation.
6. Backache or pain in legs.
7. Unbearable pain, may occur if the fibroid twists. This is a medical emergency and needs to be treated on priority basis.

Causes

Exact reason for the occurrence of fibroids might not be well understood but there are a few factors which can explain their development in the uterus.

1. **Changes in the Structure of Genes:** Many fibroids contain alterations in genes that code for uterine muscle cells. These abnormal changes in the genes might be responsible for the development of more muscle tissue and hence fibroids.

2. **Hormones:** Oestrogen and progesterone which stimulate development of the uterine lining in preparation for a possible pregnancy also appear to promote the growth of fibroids. Presence of more oestrogen receptors than normal in uterine muscle cells also point towards the role of hormones in fibroid occurrence.

3. **Other Chemicals:** Chemicals that help the body maintain tissues, such as insulin like growth factor, may affect fibroid growth.

Risk Factors

1. Being a woman of reproductive age, between puberty and menopause.
2. Heredity probably plays a role. If your mother or sister had fibroids, you are at an increased risk of also developing them.
3. Black women are not only more likely to have fibroids than women of other racial groups but their fibroids tend to occur at a younger age and are also bigger in size.
4. Obesity may be linked to the increased risk of fibroids.

Complications

1. Heavy blood loss can result in anaemia.
2. Fibroids may block the fallopian tubes and at times can hamper fertility. They can also interfere with the passage of sperms from the cervix to the fallopian tubes.
3. Pregnant women with fibroids are at a slightly increased risk of miscarriage, premature labour and delivery, abnormal foetal position and separation of the placenta from the uterine wall.
4. Rarely, the stalk of the fibroid grows out to be longer than usual and if the fibroid twists on this stalk it results in sudden, unbearable pain in the abdomen which is a medical emergency.

Diagnosis

1. **Ultrasound:** It is a safe procedure which can help diagnose fibroids. Since it does not expose a person to X-rays it can be done on pregnant women also. It takes about 20 minutes and is an outdoor procedure. You will be instructed to drink a lot of water and hold the urine before an ultrasound is done.

2. **Magnetic Resonance Imaging (MRI):** It is an expensive test and hence not done on a routine basis. This test uses powerful magnets to create a picture of the internal organs. This is also a safe investigation for pregnant women.

3. **CT Scan.**

4. **Hysteroscopy:** A thin telescope is passed into the uterus to directly look at it.

5. **Uterine X-ray:** This test is another option for diagnosing fibroids in women who are having bleeding or fertility problems. This investigation is not for pregnant women.

6. **Hysterosalpingogram (HSG).**

7. **Endometrial Biopsy:** In this test, a small piece of the uterine lining is removed and examined under a microscope. It helps in ruling out poly, cancer, infection, or any other cause of bleeding.

8. **Dilatation and Curettage (D and C):** This test allows the physician to obtain a larger piece of the lining of the uterus. It might be done instead of an endometrial biopsy if more tissue is needed or if an endometrial biopsy cannot be done.

Treatment

1. If the fibroids are asymptomatic then the doctor might just wait and watch. The patient is however called for regular medical examinations to see if the fibroid is growing further in size to rule out its chances of causing problems. The patient may be called two to three times in a year for this check up which includes an ultrasound at least once a year.

2. If the fibroid causes symptoms such as heavy bleeding then surgery is required. The two kinds of surgery most commonly performed are hysterectomy and myomectomy. In hysterectomy, the uterus is removed surgically and in myomectomy, only the fibroid is removed. The type of surgery offered to a patient depends on the size of growth. A small fibroid may be removed by a myomectomy procedure on an outpatient basis also. It may not require an abdominal surgery. The patient recovers fast and can resume daily activities quickly.

All the health care facilities as of now, are not in a situation to provide these new procedures.

   i. **Hysteroscopic Resection:** A thin telescope is inserted through the cervix into the uterus. The uterus is visualised and then the fibroid can be removed by using laser or an electrical knife. The procedure may be done with local or general anaesthesia. The woman may stay overnight in the hospital or be treated as an outpatient. Full recovery takes a week or two.

   ii. **Embolisation:** This procedure shrinks the fibroids by cutting off their blood supply. Guided by an X-ray image, the doctor puts in a catheter (a thin flexible tube) through a tiny incision in the groin into the main arteries that supply blood to the uterus. He then injects particles of inert plastic through the catheter to block these blood vessels. The uterus itself is not damaged because smaller arteries continue to supply the nutrients and oxygen it needs.

Embolisation has been used to treat fibroids in the United States for only a few years. Typically, the procedure shrinks fibroids to about half their previous size.

3. **Laparoscopic Surgery:** Some procedures can be performed using a laparoscope, a pencil-thin surgical telescope similar to a hysteroscope. The surgeon inserts the laparoscope and tiny surgical instruments through one or more small incisions in the abdomen.

Full recovery from laparoscopic surgery generally takes less than 7 days.

Fibroids and the Fear of Developing Malignancy

Most of the fibroids are not cancerous and they rarely become cancerous (leiomyosarcoma). This happens to an estimated 1 in 1,000 women who have fibroids. Some cancerous tumours may develop directly from the normal tissue in the uterus as well. The average age of women with leiomyosarcoma is 55.

Warning signs of cancer may include:

1. Rapid growth of the fibroids or the uterus.
2. Vaginal bleeding after a woman has reached menopause.

Chapter 8

Uterine Prolapse

Uterine prolapse is most commonly described when a lady says she has something coming out of the vagina.

Uterine prolapse is falling or sliding of the uterus from its normal position in the pelvic cavity into the vaginal canal (See Fig. 8.1).

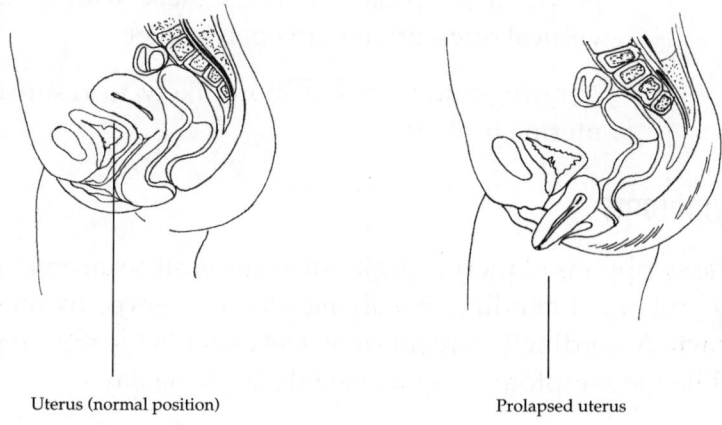

Uterus (normal position) Prolapsed uterus

Fig. 8.1: Normal and prolapsed uterus

Causes

The following conditions are associated with uterine prolapse:

1. Obstetrical trauma (increases with multiparity, size of the vaginally delivered infant) due to stretching and subsequent weakening of the pelvic support structure.

2. Congenital weakness of pelvic supports (associated with spina bifida in neonates).

3. Decreased oestrogen (as, for example, in menopause) resulting in loss of elasticity of pelvic structures.

4. Increased intra-abdominal pressure (as in obesity, chronic lung disease and asthma).

5. Certain anatomical variants are associated with an increased prevalence of uterine prolapse.

    i. Women with a wide transverse pelvic inlet appear to be at an increased risk of developing pelvic organ prolapse, as do those with a less vertical orientation of the pelvic inlet.

    ii. A retrograde uterus is more likely to result in uterine prolapse.

Symptoms

The symptoms of uterine prolapse are typically exacerbated by prolonged standing or walking and are relieved by lying down. Accordingly, patients may feel better in the morning, while the symptoms may worsen through the day.

1. Pelvic heaviness or pressure.

2. Protrusion of tissue; the patient who reports of a 'bulge' has been found to be a valuable screening tool for the detection of pelvic organ prolapse [81 per cent PPV (positive predictive value), 76 per cent NPV (negative predictive value)].
3. Pelvic pain.
4. Sexual dysfunction, including pain during sexual intercourse, decreased libido and difficulty in achieving an orgasm.
5. Low back pain.
6. Constipation.
7. Difficulty in walking.
8. Difficulty in urinating.
9. Urinary frequency increased.
10. Urinary urgency.
11. Urinary incontinence.
12. Nausea.
13. Purulent discharge (rare).
14. Bleeding (rare).

Diagnosis

A complete pelvic examination is required, including a rectovaginal examination to assess sphincter tone.

1. Physical findings may be enhanced by having the patient strain during the examination or by having her stand or walk prior to the examination. Standing with an empty bladder may result in a 1-2 stage difference in the degree of prolapse noted on examination when compared to a supine position with a full bladder.

2. Mild uterine prolapse may be recognized only when the patient strains during the bimanual examination.

3. Evaluate all patients for oestrogen status. Signs of decreased oestrogens include:
   i. Loss of rugae in the vaginal mucosa.
   ii. Decreased secretions.
   iii. Thin perineal skin.
   iv. Easy perineal tearing.

4. Physical examination should also be directed towards ruling out serious conditions that may rarely be associated with uterine prolapse, such as infection, strangulation with uterine ischaemia, urinary outflow obstruction with renal failure and haemorrhage.
   i. If urinary obstruction is present, the patient may experience tenderness over the bladder region.
   ii. If infection is present, yellow discharge from the cervix may be noted.

Treatment

Uterine prolapse can be treated with a vaginal pessary or surgery.

1. **Vaginal Pessary:** It is an object inserted into the vagina to hold the uterus in place. It may be used as a temporary or permanent form of treatment. Vaginal pessaries are fitted for each individual woman. Pessaries may cause an irritating and abnormal smelling discharge and they require periodic cleaning, usually done by the physician. In some women, they rub on and irritate the vaginal mucosa, while in some cases, the pessary may erode and cause ulcerations of the vaginal mucosal lining. Some types of pessaries may interfere

with normal sexual intercourse by limiting the depth of penetration.

If the woman is obese, attaining and maintaining optimal weight is recommended. Heavy lifting or straining should be avoided.

2. **Surgery:** Surgery should be deferred until symptoms are significant enough to outweigh the risks. Surgery, if done, usually provides excellent results. However, some women may require treatment again in the future for recurrent prolapse of the vaginal walls.

Complications

Urinary tract infections and other urinary symptoms may occur due to the frequently associated cystocoele. Constipation and haemorrhoids may also occur as a result of the associated rectocoele. Ulceration and infection may occur in more severe cases of prolapse.

Prevention

Prenatal and postpartum Kegel exercises (tightening of the pelvic floor musculature as if trying to interrupt urine flow) help to strengthen the muscles and reduces the risk (details given in chapter on urinary incontinence). Also, oestrogen replacement therapy in post-menopausal women tends to help maintain muscle tone.

Chapter 9

Dysfunctional Uterine Bleeding

Dysfunctional uterine bleeding refers to any abnormal endometrial bleeding without any known lesion or defect. It may occur in the time period between having reached menarche or before having reached menopause in a woman's reproductive life. The prognosis varies with the cause. Dysfunctional uterine bleeding is the indication for almost 25 per cent of all gynaecological surgical procedures.

Dysfunctional uterine bleeding may occur due to various causes such as:

1. When persistent stimulation of the uterus occurs due to oestrogen and there is a situation of imbalance.
2. Disorders that may cause sustained high oestrogen levels are polycystic ovary syndrome, obesity, immaturity of the hypothalamic-pituitary-ovarian mechanism.

In most of the cases, no abnormal changes can be seen under the microscope when a sample of endometrium is examined but in case the uterus keeps on getting stimulated due to exposure to oestrogen then malignant changes may be seen.

Symptoms

Dysfunctional uterine bleeding includes various symptoms such as prolonged duration of bleeding, shorter cycles and more frequent bleeding. Such uterine bleeding is unpredictable and can cause anaemia.

Treatment

1. **Drug Therapy**.
2. **Endometrial Ablation:** May be a treatment option in case children are not desired, a large portion of the bleeding endometrium is removed.
3. **Hysterectomy**.
4. **Iron and Blood:** The patient may need iron replacement or transfusions of packed cells or whole blood, as indicated, because of anaemia caused by recurrent bleeding.
5. **Hormones:** A high dose oestrogen-progesterone combination therapy may be required to control endometrial growth and reestablish a normal cyclic pattern of menstruation. You should take these drugs 4 times daily for 5-7 days, although bleeding usually stops in 12-24 hours. If the patient's age is over 35 years, endometrial biopsy is necessary before starting oestrogen therapy to rule out endometrial adenocarcinoma. Progestogen therapy is a necessary alternative in some women, such as those susceptible to the adverse effects of oestrogen.
6. **Follow up:** Regular check ups to assess the effectiveness of treatment are required.

Chapter 10

Menopause

The word menopause literally means the natural cessation of menstrual cycles, from the Greek roots 'meno-' (month) and 'pausis' (a pause, a cessation). As the life span of women increases, so will the number of women who will be achieving menopause increase. Data on the number of menopausal population is lacking in India. But still the number of women in the postmenopausal ages 50-59 years is projected to increase from 36million in 2000 to 63 million in 2020.

The normal age range for the last period is between age 45 to 55 years, with the peak being at about 51 years. If menopause is achieved between 45 to 55 years it is said to be an **'early menopause'**. And if it occurs after 55 years of age it is called **'late menopause'**. Last period prior to the age of 40 years is considered a **'premature menopause'** and this is not viewed as being due to normal causes. **'Perimenopause'** refers to the years, both before and after the last period ever, when many women find that they undergo symptoms of hormonal change and fluctuation, such as hot flashes, mood changes and insomnia. The perimenopausal period begins when there is a first break in the routine cycle.

Post-menopause is the period after having achieved menopause. Only when a woman passes 12 full months continuously without any periods, not even spotting, she is declared to have achieved menopause. The reason for this delay in declaring a woman post-menopausal is because periods become very erratic during this time; to be sure that the menstrual cycles have finally ceased, this long period is necessary.

In women who have no uterus and therefore have no periods, or in women who take certain medications because of which periods get suspended during middle age, post-menopause can be determined by a blood test which can reveal very high levels of follicle stimulating hormone typical of post-menopausal women. The average menopausal age in India is 44.3 years. Premature menopause is most common in rural areas, as well as among agricultural workers, women who are illiterate and those who have a low body-mass index. A pan-India survey, conducted recently by the Bangalore based Institute for Social and Economic Change (ISEC), highlights that on an average, nearly 4 per cent of Indian women are already menopausal between the ages of 29-34 years, one of the lowest thresholds for menopause in the world. However, women who marry and have children late do not suffer from premature menopause.

What Happens in Menopause?

During the reproductive years, a woman's ovaries produce the hormones oestrogen and progesterone. Oestrogen works to regulate a woman's monthly menstrual cycle and secondary sexual characteristics (such as breast development and function). It also rises at different times in the menstrual cycle to prepare the body for fertilisation and reproduction. Progesterone also rises in a cyclical fashion to prepare the uterus for possible pregnancy and to prepare the breasts for lactation (milk production). As a woman reaches menopause, typically around 50 years of age, her body produces less and less oestrogen and progesterone.

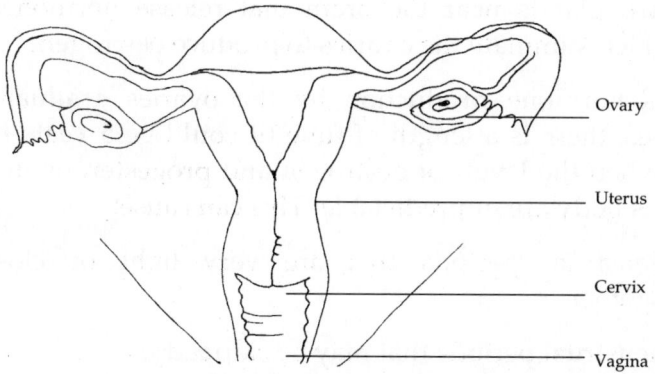

Fig. 10.1: Younger reproductive system

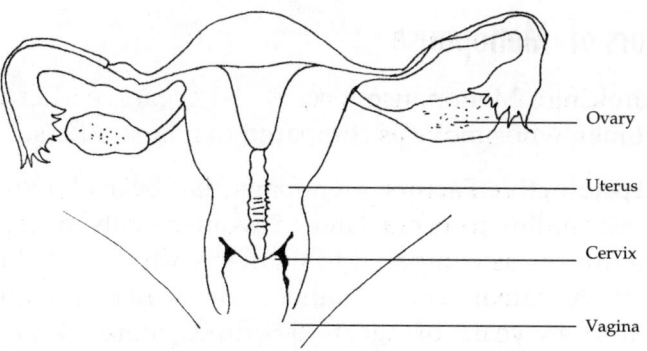

Fig. 10.2: Older reproductive system

A woman's reproductive organs include:

1. The uterus or womb.
2. Two ovaries, which produce eggs as well as the female hormones—oestrogen and progesterone (and also produce small amounts of the male hormones—testosterone and androsterone).
3. Two fallopian tubes, which transport the eggs from the ovaries to the uterus.

4. Two glands near the brain that release hormones, which stimulate the ovaries to produce oestrogen.

As hormone production by the ovaries gradually decreases, there is a length of time (it could be 5 years or more) when the levels of oestrogen and progesterone in a woman's body are unpredictable. This can cause:

1. Menstrual periods that are very light or close together.

2. Menstrual periods that may be skipped.

3. Menstrual periods that may be much heavier than usual.

Predictors of Menopause

1. **Smoking:** Menopause occurs 1-2 years earlier in women who smoke as compared to non-smokers.

2. **Reproductive Factors:** Menopause has been shown in most studies to occur later in women with multiple childbirths as compared to women with one no child birth. A woman whose mother underwent menopause before 46 years of age is 5-6 times more likely to experience menopause at an earlier age.

3. **Nutritional Factors:** Severe malnutrition can lead to earlier onset of menopause.

4. **Socio-economic Factors:** Menopause has been reported to occur later in married women of higher socio-economic class and educational background.

5. **Toxic Exposures:** Depending upon the type and location of the cancer and its treatment, these types of cancer therapy (chemotherapy and/or radiation therapy) can result in menopause if given to an

ovulating woman. In this case, the symptoms of menopause may begin during the cancer treatment or may develop in the months following the treatment.

6. **Surgical Removal of Ovaries:** The surgical removal of ovaries (oophorectomy) in an ovulating woman will result in an immediate menopause, sometimes termed as surgical menopause. In cases of surgical menopause, women often report that the abrupt onset of menopausal symptoms results in particularly severe symptoms, but this is not always the case.

    The ovaries are often removed together with the removal of the uterus (hysterectomy). If a hysterectomy is performed without removal of both ovaries in a woman who has not yet reached menopause, the remaining ovary or ovaries are still capable of normal hormone production. While a woman cannot menstruate, after the uterus is removed by hysterectomy, the ovaries themselves can continue to produce hormones until the normal time when menopause would naturally occur. At this time, a woman could experience the other symptoms of menopause like hot flashes and mood swings. These symptoms would then not be associated with the cessation of menstruation. Another possibility is that ovarian failure will occur earlier than the expected time of menopause, as early as 1-2 years following the hysterectomy. If this happens, a woman may or may not experience symptoms of menopause.

7. **Premature Ovarian Failure:** Premature ovarian failure is defined as the occurrence of menopause before the age of 40 years. This condition occurs in about 1 per cent of all women. The cause of premature ovarian failure is not fully understood, but it may be related to an autoimmune disease or genetic factors.

Symptoms

1. **Irregular Vaginal Bleeding:** Irregular vaginal bleeding may occur during menopause. Some women have minimal problems with abnormal bleeding during perimenopause whereas others have unpredictable, excessive bleeding. Menstrual periods (menses) may occur more frequently (meaning, the cycle shortens in duration), or they may get farther and farther apart (meaning the cycle lengthens in duration) before stopping. There is no 'normal' pattern of bleeding during perimenopause and patterns vary from woman to woman. It is common for women in perimenopause to get a period after going for several months without one. There is also no set length of time it takes for a woman to complete the menopausal transition. It is important to remember that all women who develop irregular menses should be evaluated by their doctor to confirm that the irregular menses are due to perimenopause and not as a sign of another medical illness.

   Menstrual abnormalities that begin in the perimenopausal period are also associated with a decrease in fertility, since ovulation becomes irregular. However, women who are in the perimenopause phase may still become pregnant until they have reached true menopause (that is, have had absence of periods continuously for one year).

2. **Hot Flashes and Night Sweats:** The symptoms of menopause vary significantly from woman to woman. Hot flashes are common among women undergoing menopause. A hot flash is a feeling of warmth that spreads over the body and is often most pronounced in the head and chest. A hot flash is sometimes associated with flushing and is sometimes followed by perspiration. Hot flashes usually last from thirty

seconds to several minutes. Although the exact cause of hot flashes is not fully understood, they occur most probably due to a combination of hormonal and biochemical fluctuations brought on by declining oestrogen levels.

There is currently no method to predict when hot flashes will begin and how long they will last. Hot flashes occur in up to 40 per cent of regularly menstruating women in their forties, so they may begin before the menstrual irregularities characteristic of menopause even begin. About 80 per cent of women will be finished having hot flashes after 5 years. Sometimes (in about 10 per cent of women) hot flashes can last as long as 10 years. There is no way to predict when hot flashes will cease, though they tend to decrease in frequency over time. On an average, hot flashes last about 5 years.

Sometimes hot flashes are accompanied by night sweats. As a result women wake up and are unable to sleep again. This can also explain why some women feel tired during the day.

Some women only experience mild menopausal symptoms while others have severe discomfort. The most common symptom of menopause is hot flashes. Hot flashes may be accompanied by sweating, flushing or heart palpitations. It is estimated that more than 60 per cent of menopausal women experience hot flashes.

3. **Vaginal Changes:** Vaginal tissue becomes thinner, drier and less elastic, which may cause discomfort or pain during sexual intercourse. Symptoms may include vaginal dryness, itching or irritation and/or pain during sexual intercourse. The vaginal changes also lead to an increased risk of vaginal infections.

4. **Urinary Tract:** Tissue of the urinary tract also becomes less elastic, which may cause a release of urine during laughter, coughing, sneezing, or exercise. Many menopausal women also find that urinary tract infections occur more frequently during this time. The lining of the urethra (the transport tube leading from the bladder to discharge urine outside the body) also undergoes changes similar to the tissues of the vagina and becomes dryer, thinner and less elastic with declining oestrogen levels. This can lead to an increased risk of urinary tract infection, feeling the need to urinate more frequently or leakage of urine (urinary incontinence). Incontinence can result from a strong, sudden urge to urinate or may occur during straining when coughing, laughing, or lifting heavy objects.

5. **Emotional and Cognitive Symptoms:** Women often report a variety of cognitive (thinking) and/or emotional symptoms, including fatigue, memory problems, irritability and rapid changes in mood. It is difficult to precisely determine exactly which behavioural symptoms are directly due to the hormonal changes of menopause. Research in this area has been difficult for many reasons. Emotional and cognitive symptoms are so common that it is sometimes difficult in a given woman to know if they are due to menopause. Night sweats that may occur can also contribute to the feeling of tiredness and fatigue, which can have an effect on mood and cognitive performance. Finally, many women may experience other life changes such as stressful life events that may also cause emotional symptoms.

Menopause

6. **Other Physical Changes:** Many women report some degree of weight gain along with menopause. The distribution of body fat may change, with body fat being deposited more in the waist and abdominal area than in the hips and thighs. Changes in skin texture, including wrinkles, may develop along with worsening of adult acne in those affected by this condition. Since the body continues to produce small levels of the male hormone testosterone, some women may experience some hair growth on the chin, upper lip, chest, or abdomen.

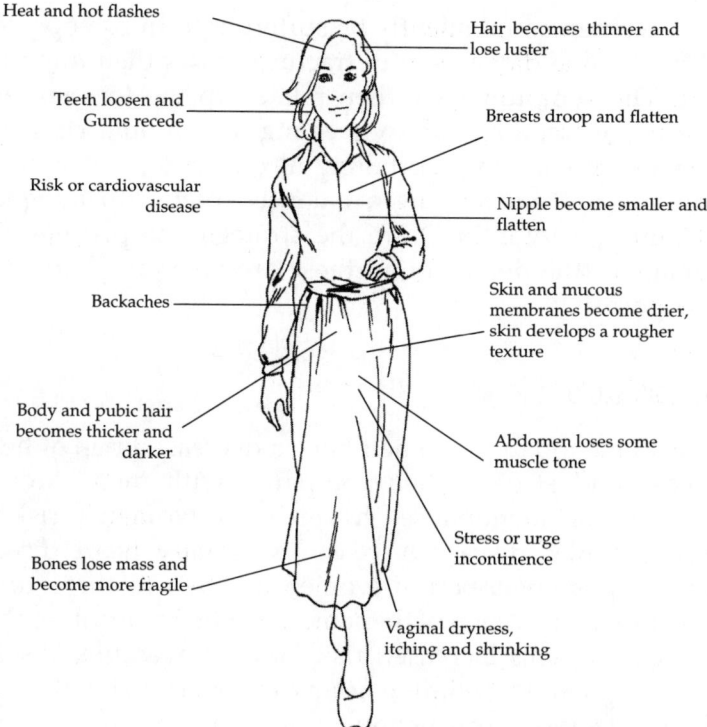

Fig. 10.3: Symptoms of menopause

Complications and Effects of Menopause on Chronic Medical Conditions

Osteoporosis

Bone density (bone mineral density) normally begins to decrease in women during the fourth decade of life. However, this normal decline in bone density is accelerated during the menopausal transition. As a consequence, both age and hormonal changes due to menopause act together to cause osteoporosis. Osteoporosis is the deterioration of the quantity and quality of bones causing an increased risk of fracture.

Women could silently be suffering from osteoporosis till finally one day a painful fracture draws their attention to it. The symptoms are then related to the location and severity of fracture. Lifestyle changes including cessation of cigarette smoking, curtailing alcohol intake, exercising regularly and consuming a balanced diet with adequate calcium and vitamin D are the strategies to prevent and manage it (the details of all these are given in chapter on osteoporosis).

Cardiovascular Disease

Prior to menopause, women have a decreased risk of heart disease and stroke when compared with men. Around the time of menopause, however, a woman's risk of cardiovascular disease increases. Coronary heart disease rates in post-menopausal women are two to three times higher than in women of the same age who have not reached menopause. This increased risk for cardiovascular disease may be related to declining oestrogen levels, but in the light of other factors, post-menopausal women are not advised to take harmone therapy simply as a preventive measure to decrease their risk of heart attack or stroke.

Self-care

Fortunately, many of the signs and symptoms associated with menopause are temporary. Take these steps to help reduce or prevent their effects:

1. **Cool Hot Flashes:** Get regular exercise, dress in layers and try to pinpoint what triggers your hot flashes. For many women, triggers may include hot beverages, spicy foods, alcohol, hot weather and even a warm room.

2. **Decrease Vaginal Discomforts:** Use over-the-counter water-based vaginal lubricants (K-Y jelly) or moisturisers. Staying sexually active also helps.

3. **Optimise Your Sleep:** Avoid caffeine and plan to exercise during the day, although not right before bedtime. Relaxation techniques, such as deep breathing, guided imagery and progressive muscle relaxation, can be very helpful. You can find a number of books and tapes on different relaxation exercises. If hot flashes disturb your sleep, you may need to find a way to manage them before you can get adequate rest.

4. **Strengthen Your Pelvic Floor:** Pelvic floor muscle exercises, called Kegel exercises, can improve some forms of urinary incontinence (details are mentioned in chapter on urinary incontinence).

5. **Eat Well:** Eat a balanced diet that includes a variety of fruits, vegetables and whole grains and that limits saturated fats, oils and sugars. Aim for 1,200 to 1,500 milligrams of calcium and 800 international units of vitamin D a day. Ask your doctor about supplements to help you meet these requirements, if necessary.

6. **Do not Smoke:** Smoking increases your risk of heart disease, stroke, osteoporosis, cancer and a range of

other health problems. It may also increase hot flashes and bring on earlier menopause. It is never too late to benefit from stopping smoking.

7. **Exercise Regularly:** Get at least thirty minutes of moderate intensity physical activity on most days to protect against cardiovascular disease, diabetes, osteoporosis and other conditions associated with aging. More vigorous exercise for longer periods may provide further benefit and is particularly important if you are trying to lose weight. Exercise can also help reduce stress.

8. **Schedule Regular Check Ups:** Talk to your doctor regarding how often you should have mammograms, pap tests, lipid level (cholesterol and triglyceride) testing and other screening tests.

Treatment

Menopause does not require any treatment as it is not a disease but a natural phenomenon that occurs in women with age. However, some of the symptoms associated with it may require intervention.

1. **Hormone Therapy:** Oestrogen therapy remains, by far, the most effective treatment option for relieving menopausal hot flashes. Depending on your personal and family medical history, your doctor may recommend oestrogen in the lowest dose needed to provide symptom relief for you.

2. **Low Dose Antidepressants.**

3. **Gabapentin (Neurontin):** Though this drug has been approved to treat seizures, it has been shown to significantly reduce hot flashes.

4. **Clonidine (Catapres, Others):** Clonidine, a pill or patch typically used to treat high blood pressure, may

significantly reduce the frequency of hot flashes, but unpleasant side effects are common.

5. **Bisphosphonates:** Doctors may recommend these non-hormonal medications which include alendronate (Fosamax), risedronate (Actonel) and ibandronate (Boniva), to prevent, or treat osteoporosis. These medications effectively reduce both bone loss and your risk of fractures and have replaced oestrogen as the main treatment for osteoporosis in women.

6. **Selective Oestrogen Receptor Modulators (SERMs):** SERMs like Raloxifene mimics oestrogen's beneficial effects on bone density in post-menopausal women, without some of the risks associated with oestrogen.

7. **Vaginal Oestrogen:** To relieve vaginal dryness, oestrogen can be administered locally using a vaginal tablet, ring, or cream. This treatment releases just a small amount of oestrogen, which is absorbed by the vaginal tissue. It can help relieve vaginal dryness, discomfort during intercourse and some urinary symptoms.

Before deciding on any form of treatment, talk to your doctor regarding your options and the risks and benefits involved with each.

Complementary and Alternative Medicine

Many approaches have been promoted as aids in managing the symptoms of menopause. Below are some complementary and alternative treatments that have been, or are being studied:

1. **Phytoestrogens:** These oestrogens occur naturally in certain foods. There are two main types of phytoestrogens—isoflavones and lignans. Isoflavones

are found in soybeans, chick peas and other legumes. Lignans occur in flax seed, whole grains and some fruits and vegetables. Researchers first became interested in phytoestrogens when they noted that women in Japan and China, who eat diets high in isoflavones, report fewer menopausal signs and symptoms and have a lower incidence of heart disease and osteoporosis than women in the West. Whether the oestrogens in these foods can relieve hot flashes and other menopausal signs and symptoms remains to be seen.

2. **Vitamin E:** This vitamin occasionally provides relief from mild hot flashes for some women. However, scientific studies have not proved its overall benefit in relieving hot flashes and taking more than 400 international units of vitamin E supplements daily may not be safe.

3. **Black Cohosh:** Black cohosh has been used widely in Europe for treating hot flashes and has been popular among women with menopausal symptoms in the United States. While its safety record has been good, there's no longer much reason to believe that it is effective for menopausal symptom relief.

You may have heard of, or even tried other dietary supplements, such as dong quai, licorice, chasteberry, evening primrose oil and wild yam (natural progesterone cream). Although some might swear by these remedies, scientific evidence of their safety and effectiveness is lacking.

Be sure to consult your doctor before taking any herbal treatment or dietary supplements for signs and symptoms of menopause. Herbal products can interfere or interact with other medications you may be taking.

Chapter 11

Hormone Replacement Therapy (HRT)

To take hormone replacement therapy or not is a question which has haunted many a women over the years. Over the past decades, women in India have perceived menopause to be a normal change associated with ageing and not taken HRT. However, now, as more and more women are getting conscious of their outwardly appearance and symptoms of menopause, they no longer want to rough it out and instead want to take HRT so that they do not suffer any problems due to decreasing levels of hormones. This has been coupled with advertising campaigns by various pharmaceutical companies who have a vested interest in promoting HRT.

What is HRT?

Hormone replacement therapy (HRT) aims to provide hormones which are depleting at the time of perimenopause. Oestrogen, progesterone and sometimes even testosterone is give to perimenopausal women from outside to restore hormonal balance in the body. It has also been used to treat women whose uterus and ovaries have been removed surgically. The symptoms of menopause and their severity vary from woman to woman. What may be appropriate for one woman may not be appropriate for another woman in terms of HRT. It is important that if you feel the need for HRT, discuss your individual case with your doctor.

HRT is available in various forms. It generally provides low dosages of one or more oestrogens and often also provides either progesterone or a progestin. Testosterone may also be included. HRT may be delivered to the body via patches, tablets, creams, IUDs, vaginal rings, gels, or more rarely, by injection. If only oestrogen is given without any progesterone, it is known as unopposed oestrogen therapy. It is usually required for women who have undergone hysterectomy. Dosage is often varied cyclically, with oestrogens taken daily and progesterone or progestins taken for about two weeks every month or two—a method called **'sequentially combined HRT'**. An alternate method, includes a constant dosage of both types of hormones daily. This method is called **'continuous combined HRT'** and is a more recent innovation. Sometimes an androgen, generally testosterone, is added to treat reduced sexual desire (libido). It may also treat reduced energy and help reduce osteoporosis after menopause. HRT is seen as either a short-term relief (often 1-2 years, usually less than 5) from menopausal symptoms hot flashes, irregular menstruation and fat redistribution) or as a longer term treatment to reduce the risk of osteopenia leading to osteoporosis. For younger women who have had their uterus or ovaries removed, usually HRT is given till the age a woman is expected to achieve menopause naturally. HRT is also used by those who have undergone a sex change procedure and aim to attain the desired secondary sexual characteristics.

What may be right for one woman may not be right for the other. So please get the initial screening done by a doctor to ascertain your suitability for starting the therapy.

The following tests are required:

1. Breast examination.
2. Internal pelvic examination.
3. Blood pressure.
4. A test for thyroid function.
5. Measurement of weight and height in order to determine Body Mass Index (BMI).
6. Mammogram.

For those who actually start taking HRT, an annual mammogram, breast examination, cervical screening and a six monthly record of blood pressure is advisable.

When to Start HRT

If a lady decides to take HRT to control her symptoms of menopause like hot flashes, vaginal dryness and itching, then she should start the therapy at the time these symptoms begin. Five years or less of HRT is considered to be safe for women. But if HRT is recommended to protect against osteoporosis then, in order to achieve maximum benefits, it should be started soon after menopause and no later than 5 years.

Side Effects of HRT

Hormone replacement therapy can cause some side effects:

Minor Side Effects

Some women who begin hormone replacement therapy experience side effects. Most of the side effects are temporary and will go away within several months. They include:

1. Bloating and fluid retention.

2. Nausea.
3. Breast tenderness (can be relieved with over-the-counter pain relievers).
4. Vaginal bleeding (may require ultrasound studies and biopsies of the tissue in the uterus).

Monthly Bleeding

When hormone replacement therapy first started, women were given oestrogen alone. This was later shown to increase their risk of certain types of cancer. In response, combination therapy was introduced, with women taking both oestrogen and progesterone.

Earlier, combination therapy caused women to bleed lightly once a month, in a fashion similar to menstrual periods, although the flow was generally lighter. Today, a new form of HRT is available that combines oestrogen and progestin. It eliminates monthly bleeding in a vast majority of women.

Hot Flashes (Vasomotor Symptoms)

Nearly 50 per cent of menopausal women have a sudden sensation of flushing and extreme warmth, followed by sweating and sometimes shaking or tremors. They occur at irregular intervals from few to many times a day.

In a Women Health Initiative Study (WHI), 10,000 post-menopausal women with a uterus were compared with a group of women whose uterus was removed by hysterectomy and were put on oestrogen and progesterone replacement therapy. The following results were revealed in the group taking hormone replacement therapy:

1. 7 more will have heart attacks.

2. 8 more will have invasive breast cancer.
3. 8 more will have stroke.
4. 18 more will have blood clots.

Trial was stopped because the risks outweighed the actual benefits of the drugs.

Protection Against Osteoporotic Fractures

WHI study confirmed reduction in osteoporotic fracture in women on combined HRT.

Psychological Symptoms

Psychological symptoms are again variable. Some women become irritable and get mood swings whereas others develop dementia and depression. There may be a decrease in sexual interest as women find themselves to be less attractive. Some women isolate themselves and withdraw themselves from routine activities. HRT can help improve these symptoms.

Genital and Breast Atrophy

At the time of menopause, many changes occur in the reproductive organs. The vagina becomes dry and itchy. Lack of lubrication leads to the complaint of pain during sexual intercourse (dyspareunia). Also, the external genital organs loose fullness. Lack of oestrogen also results in relaxation of the ligaments and hence, prolapse of uterus or urinary bladder may result. Breasts also loose their fullness and sag. Nipples become less sensitive to touch. HRT helps improve these symptoms.

Types of Therapies

In cyclic therapy, oestrogen and progesterone regimen, the progesterone must be given for a minimum of 12 days. In any case there is no place for progesterone therapy of less than 10 days duration.

In long cycle therapy that is, periods only once in 3 months or 4 times a year, progesterone must be prescribed for a minimum duration of 2 weeks and the dose of medroxyprogesterone acetate must be high that is, 20 mg daily.

Who Should Not Use HRT?

The following groups of women should not receive HRT, even if they have intolerable hot flashes:

1. Women with vaginal bleeding of unknown aetiology.
2. Breast cancer survivors.
3. Patients with active liver disease.
4. History of endometrial cancer.
5. History of venous thromboembolism.
6. Known coronary heart disease (CHD).

The following should use it cautiously, if need be:

1. Active gall bladder disease. Transdermal oestrogen preferable if decision is made to use hormonal therapy.
2. History of migraine headaches.
3. Elevated serum triglycerides (>400 mg/dl).
4. Strong family history of breast cancer (more than one first degree relative affected).

5. History of fibroids.
6. A typical ductal hyperplasia of the breast, because of substantial risk.

How HRT is Taken

0.625 mg of conjugated oestrogen Premarin is taken each day, unless you have had a hysterectomy. Progestin is also taken to decrease risk of uterine cancer. Oestrogen/progestin are available in both pill and patch form. Transdermal patch (Oestradiol 100 microgram/24 hours of estradiol). HRT daily dose gives plasma level of 200 pg/l. Hormonal therapy is given in many ways:

Continuous Combined Therapy

0.625 mg of conjugated estrogen equivalent to 5 microgram of ethinyl estradiol+10 mg of medoxy progesterone. This therapy includes fixed continuous dose of oestrogen and progestin—progestin 5 to 10 mg medroxy-progestrone for 10 to 14 days of each cycle.

Long Cycle Therapy

This therapy includes 3 months of continuous oestrogen and progesterone–progestrone for last 12 days.

American College of Obstetrics and Gynaecology, in April 2003 advocated continuous oestrogen therapy because no proven benefits in the drug-free interval were seen. Oestrogen is to be started with a low dose at 3 monthly interval. If it fails to control the symptoms, change the type of oestrogen, progesterone and also the way of delivery.

Initiating and Planning HRT Therapy

1. Perimenopausal.
2. Post-menopausal.

For therapeutic (treatment) purposes, HRT can be started at anytime provided the symptoms warrant treatment and adequate pre-therapy assessment has been performed.

For prophylaxis (to prevent symptoms of oestrogen deficiency to appear), HRT is generally started after 6-12 months of amenorrhoea, when diagnosis of menopause is certain. However, if hormone therapy has not been started at that time, it can be started in an elderly geriatric age group even in the seventh and eighth decade. However, start the therapy with a very low dose of 0.325 mg and then gradually increase to 0.625 mg after some months, if necessary.

Tibolone

Tibolone is best used in women who either have a history of breast cancer or have been treated for it as it does not stimulate the breast tissue and also does not increase the density of the breast tissue on mammogram. It causes fewer bleeding or spotting episodes and also fewer drop out rates due to bleeding. Tibolone has also been shown to increase BMD similar to that of conventional HRT. The improvement in mood and libido is superior with Tibolone. Tibolone causes a reduction in triglycerides and total cholesterol. However, it reduces HDL levels in comparison with oestrogens, which increases HDL.

Advantages of Tibolen

Tibolone is better used in patients with family history of breast cancer or treated cases on breast cancer, or who have been on conventional HRT for 5 to 10 years. Approved in 19 European countries for treatment of postmenopausal symptoms and preventing osteoporosis. It is given without progesterone. Tibolone is given without progesterone.

Disadvantages / Side Effects of Tibolen

The main disadvantages with Tibolone are reduction of HDL levels and its high cost.

Side effects include nausea in some women on initiation of therapy, but it reduces in a few weeks. Break through bleeding may also occur where patients need counselling in the first 3 months of treatment. Breast tenderness may be present but it is generally transitory. Weight gain is seen in some women. Rarely, there is an increase in hair growth because of the androgenic effect.

Herbal Remedies

As HRT is surrounded by various controversies, more and more women are taking interest in herbal remedies for management of menopause associated symptoms.

Non-HRT Modalities

1. Keeping body weight under control.
2. No smoking.
3. Avoiding alcohol.
4. Keeping cholesterol level under control.
5. Blood pressure under control.

6. Biphosphonates (Fosamax) helps against osteoporosis, another EVISTA (Raloxiphene HCL) belonging to SERMs group of drugs also protects against osteoporosis, lowers total cholesterol and prevents breast cancer.
7. Diet rich in micronutritients, multivitamins and phytoestrogens, biphosphonates and calcium.
8. Exercise.

Effect of HRT on Heart Disease and Osteoporosis

In post-menopausal women, heart disease is the leading cause of death and that is the time when the body stops producing oestrogen. Whether HRT actually decreases risk of heart disease has been a topic of much speculation. Past studies have provided hope that HRT can reduce heart disease risk. However the newer Women's Health Initiative was stopped short because the early findings showed that HRT was harmful to the heart. However women who took oestrogen and progesterone for 5 years showed less evidence of hip fracture due to osteoporosis.

Chapter 12

Urinary Incontinence

It is a condition which is common in old age and a source of embarrassment to many. When a person loses control over passage of urine, she is said to have urinary incontinence. A lady will often complain that she is not able to hold urine till she reaches the rest room and dribbling of urine occurs on the way. This situation has been often compared to that of a closed tap which leaks!

Types of Incontinence

There can be different types of incontinence:

1. **Stress Incontinence**: Whenever a person laughs sneezes, coughs, lifts weight, exercises and leakage of urine occurs, it is referred to as stress incontinence. This is the most common type of incontinence.

2. **Urge Incontinence**: The inability to hold urine long enough to reach a rest room is urge incontinence. It is often found in people who have conditions such as diabetes, stroke, dementia, Parkinson's disease and multiple sclerosis.

3. **Functional Incontinence**: When a person has another condition which creates a barrier to her reaching the rest room and leaking of urine occurs; for example, in case of osteoarthritis.

4. **Overflow Incontinence**: Leakage that occurs when the quantity of urine produced exceeds the bladder's capacity to hold it.

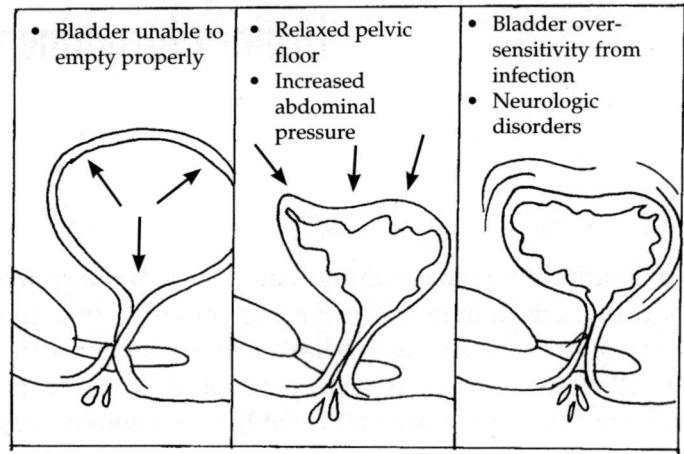

Fig. 12.1: Types of incontinence

Risk Factors

Following are some of the known factors that increase chances of urinary incontinence:

1. **Gender:** Women are more likely than men to have stress incontinence. Pregnancy and childbirth, menopause and the normal female anatomy account for this difference. However, men with prostate gland problems are at an increased risk of urge and overflow incontinence.

2. **Age:** As you grow older, the muscles of the urethra and urinary bladder become weak. As a result, ability of the bladder to hold urine decreases and chances of involuntary urine leakage increases.

3. **Obesity:** Being overweight increases the pressure on the bladder and surrounding muscles, weakening them and allowing urine to leak out when you cough or sneeze.
4. **Smoking:** A chronic cough can cause episodes of incontinence or aggravate the existing incontinence. Constant coughing puts stress on the urinary sphincter. That is a reason why smokers have a higher chance of developing incontinence.
5. **Vascular Disease:** People suffering from extensive vascular disease are at an increased risk of an overactive bladder.
6. **Participating in High Impact Sports:** High impact sports such as running, basketball and gymnastics can cause episodes of incontinence in otherwise healthy women. These vigorous activities put sudden, strong pressure on your bladder, allowing urine to leak past your urinary sphincter. But whether it leads to chronic incontinence is still not clear.
7. **Other Diseases:** Having kidney disease or diabetes may increase the risk of urinary incontinence.

Symptoms

The following are the most common symptoms of urinary incontinence. What may be the presentation in one individual may not be the case with another.

1. Inability to urinate or pain related to urination without an existing infection of the bladder.
2. Progressive weakness of the urinary stream with or without a feeling of incomplete bladder emptying.
3. Increase in frequency of urination that is, a person goes more number of times to the rest room to pass urine.

4. Loosing control over urination; as a result one rushes to the rest room to pass urine.
5. A person with spinal cord injury, stroke, etc. finds a change in her urination pattern.
6. A person restricts her activities on account of leakage of urine.
7. After a surgical procedure is performed, the lady develops urination related problem.
8. Frequent episodes of bladder infection.

Diagnosis

For people with urinary incontinence, it is important to consult a physician for a complete physical examination that focuses on the urinary and nervous systems, reproductive organs and urine samples. Many of these patients are finally referred to urologists.

Treatment

Specific treatment for urinary incontinence will be determined by your physician based on your age, overall health, medical history and extent of disease. Your tolerance for specific medications, procedures or therapies is also considered.

Treatment may include:

1. Certain behavioural techniques (including pelvic muscle exercises, biofeedback and bladder training).
2. Medications.
3. Surgery.
4. Diet modifications (including eliminating caffeine in coffee, soda and tea and/or eliminating alcohol).

Management

Since incontinence affects you physically as well as leads to embarrassment, you should definitely try and get treatment. Please do not feel shy and ignore the problem. Depending on the cause, treatment is provided. Hence, there are very many ways of treat it. What is most appropriate for you is to be decided by your doctor after a full evaluation at an individual basis.

Following interventions may be helpful in controlling incontinence:

1. **Lifestyle Changes:** Many bladder problems can be significantly improved by making changes to the patient's lifestyle or home environment. These might include changes in diet, voiding schedules or prompting from a family member or caretaker to make it easier for a patient to get to the bathroom.

2. **Biofeedback:** Biofeedback training is commonly used to teach patients how to locate, learn to exercise and control their pelvic floor muscles. After a short training session at the clinic, most patients feel comfortable about doing their pelvic muscle exercises at home. In a biofeedback session, a nurse, therapist or technician will either insert a monitoring probe into your vagina or place adhesive electrodes on the skin outside your vagina or rectal area. When you contract your pelvic floor muscles, you'll see a measurement on a monitor that lets you know whether you've successfully contracted the right muscles. You'll also be able to see how long you hold the contraction.

   Later, you'll probably be able to duplicate the exercise on your own. Because simpler methods work for most women, this technique is rarely used.

3. **Electrical Stimulation:** This is a battery powered device that stimulates the muscles around the urethra, making them stronger and tighter. The unit is pre-set for each individual and the patient uses it either at home or at the clinic.

4. **Medications:** There are several medications that can help urinary incontinence, including those that calm overactive bladders and those that tighten the bladder outlet.

5. **Pelvic Muscle Exercises:** These exercises are designed to strengthen the pelvic floor muscles to help prevent urine loss and also to help calm an overactive bladder.

    i. **Kegel Exercises:** These exercises are specifically designed to strengthen the urinary muscles. To do them, tighten your muscles as if you are trying to stop urination or trying not to pass gas. Doing 20 repetitions of this exercise, morning and night can help to control incontinence.

    Kegel is the name of a pelvic floor exercise, named after Dr Kegel who discovered the exercise. The muscles are attached to the pelvic bone and act like a hammock, holding your pelvic organs. To try and isolate these muscles, try stopping and starting the flow of urine.

    Kegeling provides many benefits:

    a. Conditioned muscles will make the process of giving birth easier and your perineum will more likely be intact (that is, have fewer tears and episiotomies) after delivery.

    b. Sexual enjoyment is enhanced for both partners.

Urinary Incontinence

c. It can prevent prolapse of pelvic organs.

d. It helps prevent leakage of urine when you sneeze or cough.

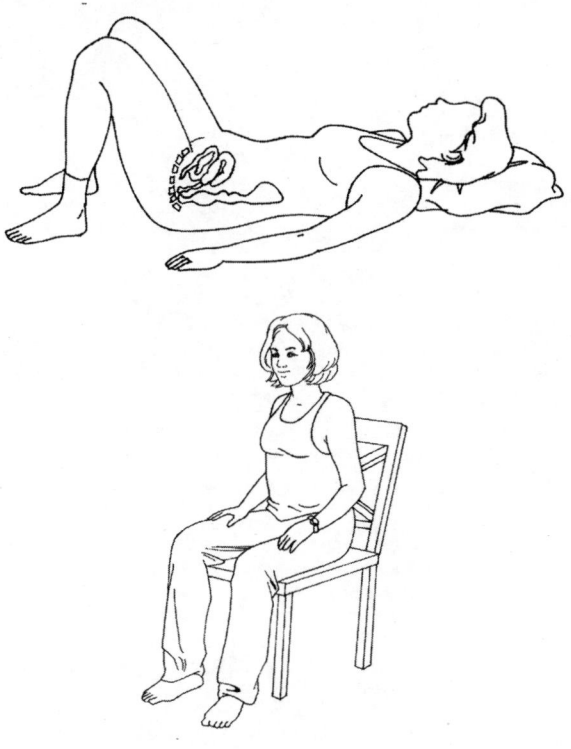

Fig. 12.2: Kegel's exercises

Now-a-days, adult diapers are available in the market which a person can use without discomfort to avoid embarrassment. Also, to provide an outlet to the urine, a catheter can also be inserted into the urethra.

As we grow older, the problem of incontinence is likely to become common, but if we prepare ourselves in the earlier part of life and take adequate precautions there is a good chance that it can be controlled.

Chapter 13

Hypertension (High Blood Pressure)

High blood pressure is one entity we all are aware of. This condition usually develops gradually over a period of time and is more common in the older age group. Blood pressure is determined by the amount of blood your heart pumps and the amount of resistance provided to the blood flow in your arteries. The more blood your heart pumps and the narrower your arteries, the higher your blood pressure is. A blood pressure reading, given in millimeters of mercury (mm of Hg), has two numbers. The first or upper number measures the pressure in your arteries when your heart beats (systolic pressure). The second or lower number measures the pressure in your arteries between beats (diastolic pressure).

For most of us, a blood pressure reading of 120/ 80 mm of Hg is considered to be normal. Both numbers in a blood pressure reading are important. However, after the age of 50, the systolic reading is more significant. When the diastolic pressure is normal but the systolic pressure is high, the condition is known as **isolated systolic hypertension** and this is fairly common in those above 50 years of age.

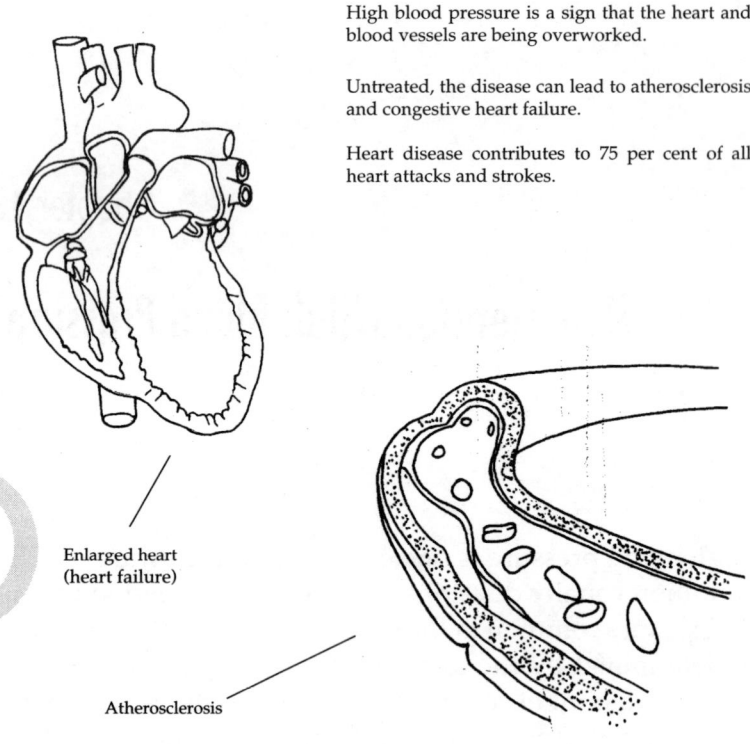

Fig. 14.1: High blood pressure

High blood pressure is a sign that the heart and blood vessels are being overworked.

Untreated, the disease can lead to atherosclerosis and congestive heart failure.

Heart disease contributes to 75 per cent of all heart attacks and strokes.

Usually three blood pressure readings, each at two or more separate appointments are taken before diagnosing hypertension. You can also record the blood pressure at home and show the records to your doctor. The reason is, when you go to see your doctor you may develop **white coat hypertension**. Also, blood pressure varies through the day.

Risk Factors

High blood pressure has many risk factors.

Unmodifiable High Risk Factors for Hypertension

1. **Age:** The risk of high blood pressure increases as you age. Through early middle age, high blood pressure is more common in men. Women are more likely to develop high blood pressure after menopause.

2. **Race:** High blood pressure is particularly common among blacks, often developing at an earlier age than in whites. Serious complications, such as stroke and heart attack, are also more common in blacks.

3. **Family History:** High blood pressure tends to run in families.

Modifiable High Risk Factors

1. **Being Overweight or Obese:** The more you weigh, the more blood you need to supply oxygen and nutrients to your tissues. As the volume of blood circulated through your blood vessels increases, so does the pressure on your artery walls.

2. **Not Being Physically Active:** People who are inactive tend to have higher heart rates. The higher your heart rate, the harder your heart must work with each contraction and the stronger the force on your arteries. Lack of physical activity also increases the risk of being overweight.

3. **Using Tobacco:** Not only does smoking tobacco immediately raise your blood pressure temporarily, but the chemicals in tobacco can damage the lining of your artery walls. This can cause your arteries to narrow, further increasing your blood pressure.

4. **Too Much Salt (Sodium) in Your Diet:** Too much sodium in your diet can cause your body to retain fluid, which increases blood pressure.

5. **Too Little Potassium in Your Diet:** Potassium helps balance the amount of sodium in your cells. If you do not consume or retain enough potassium, you may accumulate too much sodium in your blood.

6. **Drinking Too Much Alcohol:** Over time, heavy drinking can damage your heart. Having more than two or three drinks in one sitting can also temporarily raise your blood pressure, as it may cause your body to release hormones that increase your blood flow and heart rate.

7. **Stress:** High levels of stress can lead to a temporary, but dramatic, increase in blood pressure. If you try to relax by eating more, using tobacco or drinking alcohol, you may only increase problems with high blood pressure.

8. **Other Conditions:** Other conditions like high cholesterol, diabetes, kidney disease and sleep apnoea also contribute towards hypertension. Sometimes pregnancy contributes to high blood pressure as well.

Symptoms

Most people with high blood pressure have no signs or symptoms, even if blood pressure readings reach dangerously high levels.

Although a few people with early stage high blood pressure may have dull headaches, dizzy spells or a few more nosebleeds than normal, these signs and symptoms typically do not occur until high blood pressure has reached an advanced stage.

Types

There are two types of high blood pressure. When hypertension develops without any identifiable cause it is known as **essential** or **primary hypertension**. This accounts for 90 to 95 per cent of the cases in adults. In 5 to 10 per cent hypertension cases, it tends to appear suddenly and cause higher blood pressure than primary hypertension. This is known as **secondary hypertension**. Various medications and conditions like kidney abnormalities, tumours of the adrenal gland, congenital heart disease, oral contraceptive pills, illegal drugs like cocaine and without prescription drugs like amphetamines are the underlying cause for it.

Measuring Your Blood Pressure at Home

Some people are asked by their doctor to measure their blood pressure at home to find out the actual readings minus the stress of sitting in a clinic or presence of a doctor. This is called **white coat hypertension** and can be caused by feeling anxious, or by being in a busy or noisy environment. This can affect readings by as much as 30 mm of Hg (systolic reading). For those already on treatment for hypertension, monitoring blood pressure over a period of time at home can also provide your doctor or nurse with more information about how well your treatment is working and how you respond to medications. Home blood pressure monitoring can also be useful for people who have high blood pressure and who are taking medications as it can mean that you are able to cut down on the number of visits to your surgery for checks.

What do your blood pressure numbers mean/

Blood pressure is measured by two numvbers.

Systolic pressure
120
80
Diastolic pressure

Your provider will read this blood pressure as '120 over 80'

The first (or top) number 'systolic'—is the pressure in your blood vessels when your heart beats. The second (or bottom) number—'diastolic'—is the pressure in your blood vessels between heartbeats.

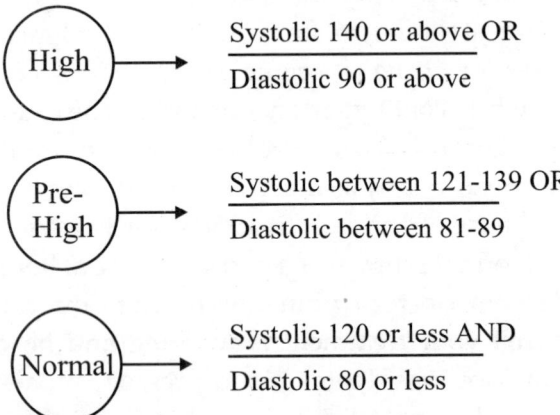

(High) → Systolic 140 or above OR / Diastolic 90 or above

(Pre-High) → Systolic between 121-139 OR / Diastolic between 81-89

(Normal) → Systolic 120 or less AND / Diastolic 80 or less

Choosing a Blood Pressure Monitor

Aneroid Monitor

One advantage of the aneroid monitor is that it can easily be carried from one place to another. Also, the cuff for the device has a built-in stethoscope, so you do not need to buy a separate stethoscope. It's also easier to manage this way. The unit may have a special feature that makes it easier to put the cuff on with one hand. In addition, the aneroid monitor costs less than digital monitors. The aneroid monitor also has some disadvantages. First, it is a complicated device that can easily be damaged and become less accurate. The device is also difficult to use if it does not have the special feature—a metal ring—that makes it easier to put the cuff on. In addition, the rubber bulb that inflates the cuff may be difficult to squeeze. This monitor may not be appropriate for hearing-impaired people, because of the need to listen to heart sounds through the stethoscope.

Steps Involved in Using an Aneroid Monitor

1. Put the stethoscope ear pieces into your ears, with the ear pieces facing forward.
2. Place the stethoscope disk on the inner side of the crease of your elbow.
3. Rapidly inflate the cuff by squeezing the rubber bulb 30 to 40 points higher than your last systolic reading. Inflate the cuff rapidly, not just a little at a time. Inflating the cuff too slowly will cause a false reading.
4. Slightly loosen the valve and slowly let some air out of the cuff. Deflate the cuff by 2 to 3 millimeters per second. If you loosen the valve too much, you won't be able to determine your blood pressure.
5. As you let the air out of the cuff, you will begin to hear the heartbeat. Listen carefully for the first sound. Check the blood pressure reading by looking at the pointer on the dial. This number will be your systolic pressure.

6. Continue to deflate the cuff. Listen to your heartbeat. You will hear your heartbeat stop at some point. Check the reading on the dial. This number is your diastolic pressure.
7. Write down your blood pressure, putting the systolic pressure before the diastolic pressure (for example, 120/80).

If you want to repeat the measurement, wait two to three minutes before reinflating the cuff.

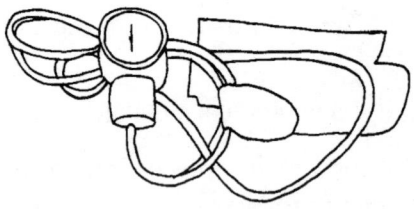

Fig. 13.1: Aneroid blood pressure monitor

Digital Monitor

Digital monitor is automatic and hence it is the most popular blood pressure measuring device. The blood pressure measurement is easy to read, because the numbers are shown on a screen. Some electronic monitors have a paper printout that gives you a record of the blood pressure reading.

It has a gauge and stethoscope that are one unit and the numbers are easy to read. It also has an error indicator and deflation is automatic. Inflation of the cuff is either automatic or manual, depending upon the model. This blood pressure monitoring device is good for hearing-impaired patients, since there is no need to listen to heart sounds through the stethoscope.

A disadvantage of the digital monitor is that the accuracy is changed by body movements or an irregular heart rate. In addition, the monitor requires batteries. However, the device is very easy to use. Just put the cuff around the arm, turn the power on and start the machine.

Steps Involved in Using a Digital Monitor

1. The cuff will inflate by itself with a push of a button on the automatic models. On the semiautomatic models, the cuff is inflated by squeezing the rubber bulb. After the cuff is inflated, the automatic mechanism will slowly reduce the cuff pressure.

2. Look at the display window to see your blood pressure reading. The machine will show your systolic and diastolic blood pressures on the screen. Write down your blood pressure, putting the systolic pressure before the diastolic pressure.

3. Press the exhaust button to release all the air from the cuff.

4. If you want to repeat the measurement, wait 2 to 3 minutes before reinflating the cuff.

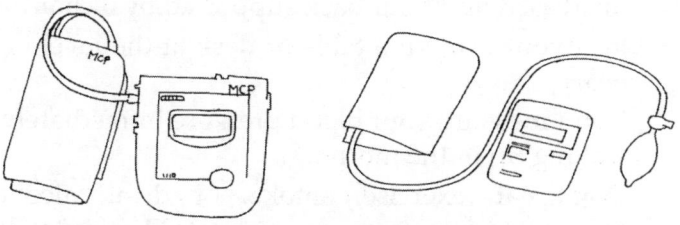

Fig. 13.2: Digital fully automatic   Fig. 13.3: Digital semiautomatic

Normal blood pressure is 120/80 mm of Hg or lower. High blood pressure is 140/90 mm of Hg or higher. The excessive pressure on your artery walls caused by high blood pressure can damage your blood vessels, as well as organs in the body. The higher your blood pressure and the longer it goes uncontrolled, the greater the damage.

The first priority when buying a monitor is to choose one that you know is accurate. So:

1. Choose a machine that measures from the top of the arm, rather than the wrist or the finger. Finger monitors will not give accurate readings and wrist monitors are also less likely than upper arm monitors to give an accurate reading.
2. The right size of cuff is important for an accurate reading. 4 out of every 5 people are able to use the standard size cuff that comes with the monitor and get an accurate reading. However, some people have very thin or very large arms and a standard size cuff may produce inaccurate readings. If the cuff is too small, the reading may be falsely high and if it is too big, the reading may be falsely low.
3. Measure your blood pressure several times a day at the same time each day because blood pressures vary throughout the day.
4. Get duplicate readings separated by 2 - 3 minutes.
5. Before you measure blood pressure, sit quietly and comfortably for about 5 minutes with your legs uncrossed and your back supported by a chair.
6. Rest your arm on a table or desk at the level of your heart.
7. Don't measure your blood pressure immediately after waking up in the morning.
8. Don't eat, exercise, smoke, or drink alcohol or caffeinated beverages for at least 30 minutes before taking your blood pressure.
9. Use the same arm each time you check your blood pressure.

Measuring Blood Pressure the Right Way

Preparation

1. Calm, warm environment.
2. No exercising in the preceding 30 min.
3. No coffee, food, smoking or decongestant in the preceding hour.
4. Empty bladder and bowel.
5. Patient calmly seated for five minutes.

Device

1. Validated device.
2. Have the device calibrated regularly according to manufacturers' recommendations.
3. Cuff size: small, medium, or large according to arm size.

Home BP Measurement

1. Two measurments morning and evening for 7 days.
2. Discard measurements of day 1.
3. Average the numbers.

Target Value

1. Below 135/85 mmHg.
2. Office BP Measurement.
3. Two measurements; same arm, same position.
4. Average the numbers.
5. Do not round the numbers.

Target Value

1. < 140/90 mmHg.
2. < 130/80 mmHg diabetes or nephropathy.

Aspects to be taken care of

1. Do not speak.
2. Keep back supported.
3. Place cuffed arm at heart level.
4. Keep legs uncrossed.
5. Be seated.
6. Keep feet flat on the floor.
7. Place cuff 3 cm from the fold of the elbow.
8. Ensure arm is supported.

However, if you find that on repeated measurements your blood pressure over a period of time is higher than usual, go and see your doctor or nurse, taking details of the measurements with you. The important readings are the averages over a period of time and not individual readings.

Low Blood Pressure

We have often heard ladies complain about the problem of low blood pressure. But what is this entity and does it actually exist? Hypotension or low blood pressure, happens when your systolic pressure is consistently (several blood pressure readings over several days) below 90, or 25 points below your normal reading. Hypotension can be a sign of something serious such as shock or a life threatening condition. Contact your doctor immediately if you are dizzy or fainting.

Other Investigations

If you have any type of high blood pressure, your doctor may recommend routine tests, such as a urine test (urinalysis), blood tests and an electrocardiogram (ECG)—a test that measures your heart's electrical activity.

Prevention and Control

Lifestyle changes can help you control and prevent high blood pressure.

1. Eat healthy foods. Try the Dietary Approaches to Stop Hypertension (DASH) diet, which emphasises fruits, vegetables, whole grains and low fat dairy foods. Get plenty of potassium, which can help prevent and control high blood pressure. Eat less saturated fat and total fat.
2. Decrease the salt in your diet. Although 2,400 mg of sodium a day is the current limit for otherwise

healthy adults, limiting sodium intake to 1,500 mg a day will have a more dramatic effect on your blood pressure. While you can reduce the amount of salt you eat by putting down the saltshaker, you should also pay attention to the amount of salt that's in the processed foods you eat, such as canned soups or frozen dinners.
3. Maintain a healthy weight. If you are overweight, losing even 5 pounds (2.3 kilograms) can lower your blood pressure.
4. Increase physical activity. Regular physical activity can help lower your blood pressure and keep your weight under control. Strive for at least 30 minutes of physical activity a day.
5. Limit alcohol. Even if you are healthy, alcohol can raise your blood pressure. If you choose to drink alcohol, do so in moderation—up to one drink a day for women and everyone over the age of 65 years and two drinks a day for men.
6. Don't smoke. Tobacco injures blood vessel walls and speeds up the process of hardening of the arteries. If you smoke, ask your doctor to help you quit.
7. Manage stress. Reduce stress as much as possible. Practice healthy coping techniques, such as muscle relaxation and deep breathing. Getting plenty of sleep can help too.
8. Monitor your blood pressure at home. Home blood pressure monitoring can help you keep closer tabs on your blood pressure, show if medication is working and even alert you and your doctor to potential complications. If your blood pressure is under control, you may be able to make fewer visits to your doctor if you monitor your blood pressure at home.
9. Practice relaxation or slow, deep breathing. Do it on your own or try a device-guided paced breathing.

Chapter 14

Diabetes

Diabetes affects over 150 million people worldwide and this number is expected to double by 2025.

It is type II diabetes which is more common in older women, especially if they are obese as well. In this type there is a problem with the cells that respond to insulin rather than production of insulin which is the case with type

1. When the body does not have enough insulin or cannot use insulin properly, sugar cannot get into your cells. Sugar builds up in your blood and it is this build up of sugar in your blood if not controlled, that leads to complications.

Some individuals suffer from a condition known as **pre-diabetes,** in which your blood sugar level is higher than normal, but not high enough to be classified as type 2 diabetes. Pre-diabetes is likely to become type 2 diabetes in as little as 10 years. However, healthy lifestyle changes along with proper treatment can control your blood sugar level.

Causes of Diabetes

1. Exact cause is not known.
2. Obesity.
3. Lack of physical exercise.
4. Family history of diabetes mellitus.
5. Those with diabetes during pregnancy that is, gestational diabetes.
6. Menopause may also contribute to diabetes. Diabetes and menopause together can have varied effects on your body. The hormones, oestrogen and progesterone affect how your cells respond to insulin. During menopause, changes in your hormone levels can trigger fluctuations in your blood sugar level. Some weight gain also occurs during menopause which contributes towards diabetes. Diabetes makes a person more prone to infections but after menopause the situation worsens as the level of oestrogen drops, making it easier for disease organisms to cause infection in the urinary tract and vagina. Sexual arousal is also decreased as cells lining the wall of the vagina are damaged and the vagina becomes dry also.

Symptoms of Adult Type 2 Diabetes

1. Increased frequency of passing urine.
2. Increased thirst.
3. Increased appetite.
4. Unexpected weight gain or weight loss.
5. Blurred vision.
6. Skin infections.
7. Vaginal infections.
8. Tiredness
9. Slowly healing sores / wounds.

10. Abnormal feelings of prickling, burning or itching of the skin, usually on the hands or feet.

Diagnosis

Two blood tests may be done to diagnose type 2 Diabetes:

1. **Fasting Blood Sugar (FBS):** A sample of your blood is tested in the morning before you have eaten anything. If this test shows you have a fasting blood sugar of

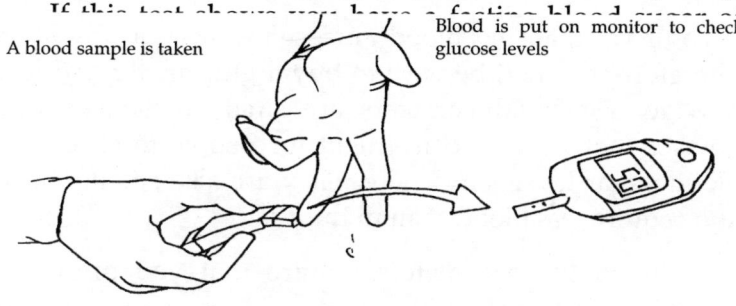

A blood sample is taken

Blood is put on monitor to check glucose levels

Fig. 14.2: Blood glucose testing

126 milligrams per deciliter (mg/dL) or more, you may be diabetic. Often a second test will be done after you have fasted since your evening meal and all night. If this second test confirms your high blood sugar, diagnosis of diabetes is made.

2. **Oral Glucose Tolerance Test (OGTT):** For the glucose tolerance test, a sample of your blood is taken when you have not eaten anything since the night before. Then you drink a special high sugar drink and your blood is tested 2 hours again later. If after 2 hours your blood sugar level is 200 mg/dL or higher, you are diabetic.

The World Health Organization definition of diabetes is for a single raised glucose reading with symptoms, otherwise raised values on two occasions, of either – fasting plasma glucose 7.0 mmol/l (126 mg/dl) or with a glucose tolerance test, 2 hours after the oral dose a plasma glucose š 11.1 mmol/l (200 mg/dl).

Help Yourself

Self-testing of Blood Glucose

If you have diabetes, blood glucose testing is a way of life. Therefore it would be wise to buy a glucometer and learn how to use it. Glucometers are small, battery-operated devices that make it convenient for people to check their blood sugar levels anywhere. They are also smaller, faster and require less blood than in the past.

Blood glucose meters require that you prick your finger or an alternative site and put a drop of blood on a test strip that is inserted into the meter.

Benefits of Testing at Home

1. Testing regularly allows you to look for patterns to see if your blood glucose is in a safe range. If not, a change in diet, increase in exercise or a visit to your healthcare provider for medication to lower blood sugar and your risk of complications may be needed.
2. Blood glucose monitoring can also tell you if your blood sugar is too low, a potentially dangerous situation that requires you to eat or drink something with 10-15 grams of carbohydrates.

   You have probably seen many advertisements for blood glucose meters and are wondering which meter is the best one for you. Most meters are accurate in how they measure your glucose but they differ in type and number of features that they offer.

i. Before buying a meter, check the cost of a meter test strip. A meter may be the cheapest one on the market, but it is not a good deal if the strips costs twice as much.
ii. Size of the glucometer matters to the patient. Small meters are more convenient for carrying, but also require more dexterity to use.
iii. Look at the packaging for the test strips. If you have vision problems, look for a meter with a larger display, or voice module.
iv. Blood sample size is also to be considered. Check to see how big a blood sample is needed for blood glucose testing. Blood sample size ranges from 0.3 (amount that would fit on the head of a pin) to 4.0 microliters.
v. Check during the night. Consider a meter that has a backlight.

When to Test Your Blood Sugar

How often you need to test your blood sugar level depends on the type of diabetes you have and your individual diabetes treatment plan.

If you have type 1 diabetes, your doctor may recommend testing your blood sugar level at least three times a day—perhaps before and after certain meals, before and after exercise and before bed. You may need to check your blood sugar level more often if you are ill or you change your daily routine.

If you take medication—with or without insulin—to manage type 2 diabetes, your doctor may recommend testing your blood sugar level once a day. If you manage type 2 diabetes with diet and exercise alone, you may need to test your blood sugar level even less often.

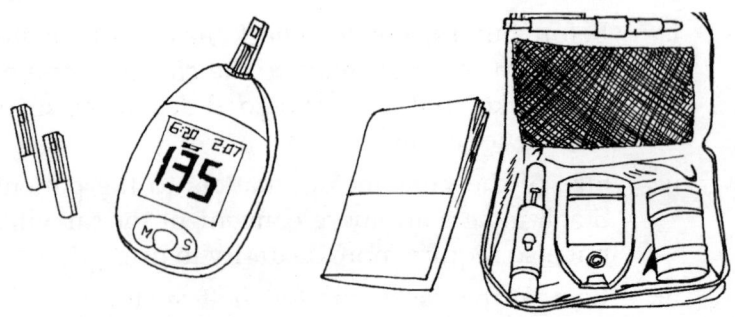

Fig. 14.3: Glucometer

How to Test Your Blood Sugar at Home

To test your blood sugar level, you'll need a blood sugar monitor. Some monitors are large with easy-to-handle test strips, while others are compact and easier to carry. Some monitors track the time and date of each test, the result and trends over time.

Most blood sugar monitors require you to prick your fingertip with a special needle (lancet).

If you wonder which type of blood sugar monitor would be best for you, ask your doctor or diabetes educator for a recommendation.

When used correctly, you can count on your blood sugar monitor to provide accurate readings. If you think something's not right, start with the basics:

1. Check the test strips. Throw out damaged or outdated strips.

2. Check the monitor. Make sure the monitor is at room temperature and the strip guide and the test window are clean. Replace the batteries in the monitor, if needed.

3. Check the measurement scale (calibration). Some

monitors must be calibrated to each container of test strips. Be sure the code number in the monitor matches the code number on the container of test strips.

4. Check your technique. Wash your hands with soap and water before pricking your finger. Apply a generous drop of blood to the test strip. Do not add more blood to the test strip after the first drop was applied.

5. You can bring the monitor to your next doctor's appointment as well.

1. Gather Your Tools

Blood sugar testing is usually done with a special needle called a lancet and an electronic glucose monitor. Start by gathering your supplies:

i. Lancet.

ii. Lancing device cap for finger sticks.

iii. Lancing device cap for alternate-site sticks.

iv. Glucose monitor.

v. Lancing device.

vi. Dial to set depth of skin puncture (available on some lancing devices).

vii. Vial containing test strips.

viii. Test strip.

2. Code Your Meter

Some glucose monitors must be coded every time you open a new vial of test strips. Each meter has its own coding technique. Follow the manufacturer's instructions carefully. Be sure to keep the instructions handy for future reference.

Some meters have a code chip—often called a key—that slips into the device. In this image, the code number on the vial of test strips has been entered into the monitor using the button labelled 'C'.

Some newer monitors do not need coding.

3. Wash Your Hands

Wash your hands with soap and warm water. Dry them completely. If you do not have access to soap and warm water, use an alcohol pad to clean the area you plan to stick. Because alcohol can affect your blood sugar reading, dry the area completely before pricking your skin.

4. Prick Your Fingertip

Before you prick your fingertip, load the test strip into your meter. If you are using a lancing device similar to the one shown here, make sure you've attached the lancing tip for finger pricks. It's usually opaque.

Use the depth dial on the top of the lancing device to select the penetration depth of your lancing tip. Place the tip covering the lancet on the side of your fingertip, which is less sensitive than the flat side of the tip of your finger. Press the button to discharge the lancet.

5. Hold the Lancing Device Cap Down

Press the lancing device cap down until you have a drop of blood that's large enough to test.

Don't use an alternate site for testing if you think your blood sugar level is low, if you've just eaten or taken medication, or you've just exercised. Blood samples from alternate sites are not as accurate as fingertip samples when your blood sugar level is rising or falling quickly.

6. Record Your Results

Record the results of each blood sugar test.

7. Discard Your Lancet

Place the used lancet in a safe container. When the container is full, ask your waste management company regarding proper disposal. Containers with used lancets are considered hazardous waste.

8. Store Your Equipment

Take special care to keep your equipment out of hot or cold places, such as the glove compartment in your car in summer or winter. When you travel, place your medication prescription with your glucose testing kit. Carry these items with you.

How to Maintain Your Blood Sugar Level Steady

Food

1. Be consistent with food. Your blood sugar level is highest an hour or two after you eat and then begins to fall. But this predictable pattern can work to your advantage. Simply eating about the same amount of food at about the same time every day can help you control your blood sugar level.

    Don't eat too many carbohydrates at one go. Carbohydrates have a bigger impact on your blood sugar level than proteins or fats. Eating about the same amount of carbohydrates at each meal or snack will help keep your blood sugar level steady throughout the day.

Coordinate your meals and medication. Too little food in comparison to your diabetes medications, especially insulin, may result in dangerously low blood sugar (hypoglycaemia). Too much food may cause your blood sugar level to climb too high (hyperglycaemia). Your diabetes health care team can help you strike a balance.

The key to diabetes nutrition is moderation.

Total amount of carbohydrate consumed is what counts. As long as the sweets are taken with a meal and balanced with other foods in your meal plan, they can be consumed. It is the total amount of carbohydrate that counts the most.

If you have diabetes, you should follow these guidelines when making food choices:

i. **Carbohydrates:** Between 45 per cent and 65 per cent of your daily calories should come from carbohydrates.

ii. **Fat:** No more than 20 per cent to 35 per cent of your total daily calories should come from fats. Of those calories, no more than 7 per cent should come from saturated fat and you should try to avoid all trans fat.

iii. **Protein:** Between 15 per cent and 20 per cent of your total daily calories should come from proteins.

iv. **Cholesterol:** Limit cholesterol to less than 200 mg a day.

Some people with diabetes use the glycaemic index (GI) as a guide in selecting foods, especially carbohydrates—for meal planning. The glycaemic index ranks carbohydrate-containing foods based on their effect on blood sugar level. Foods with a high glycaemic-index value tend to raise your blood sugar faster and higher than do foods with a lower value.

Although the glycaemic index diet has some potential benefits such as reducing blood sugar levels it is very complicated.

Exercise

Physical activity is another important part of your diabetes management plan. When you exercise, your muscles use sugar (glucose) for energy. Regular physical activity also improves your body's response to insulin. These factors work together to lower your blood sugar levels. The more strenuous your workout, the longer the effect lasts. But even light activities such as housework, gardening or being on your feet for extended periods can lower your blood sugar levels. Exercise good judgment. Check your blood sugar level before, during and after exercise, especially if you take insulin or medications that can cause low blood sugar. Drink plenty of fluids while you work out. Stop exercising if you experience any warning signs, such as severe shortness of breath, dizziness or chest pain.

Medication

Insulin and other diabetes medications are designed to lower your blood sugar level. However, the effectiveness of these medications depends on the timing and size of the dose. Any medication you take for conditions other than diabetes can also affect your blood sugar levels.

Illness

When you are sick, your body produces hormones to help fight the illness. These hormones raise your blood sugar level by preventing insulin from working effectively. You should have a special plan framed for sickness.

Alcohol

The liver normally releases stored sugar to counteract falling blood sugar levels. But if your liver is busy metabolising alcohol, your blood sugar level may not get the boost it needs. If you take insulin or oral diabetes medications, even as little as 2 ounces of alcohol—the equivalent of two drinks can cause low blood sugar.

Alcohol can aggravate diabetic complications, such as nerve damage and eye disease. But if your diabetes is under control and your doctor agrees, an occasional alcoholic drink with a meal is fine.

Remember to include the calories from any alcohol you drink in your daily calorie count.

Hormone Levels

As your hormonal levels fluctuate during your menstrual cycle, so can your blood sugar levels, particularly in the week before your period. Menopause may trigger fluctuations in your blood sugar level as well.

Stress

Under stress, it is not easy to stick to a healthy plan that is, eating on time and exercising as per the schedule. You should learn to distress yourself and prioritize your tasks.

Watch Out for Fall in Blood Glucose Levels

Hypoglycaemia, often defined as blood sugar below 70 mg/dL or 4 millimoles per liter (mmol/L) occurs when there's too much insulin and not enough sugar (glucose) in your blood. Hypoglycaemia is most common among people who take insulin, but it can also occur if you are taking oral diabetic medication.

Culprits may include:

1. Taking too much diabetes medication.
2. Not eating enough.
3. Postponing or skipping a meal.
4. Increasing physical activity without eating more.
5. Drinking alcohol.

Paying attention to the early signs and symptoms of hypoglycaemia can help you treat the condition promptly. Early danger signs include:

1. Shakiness.
2. Clumsiness.
3. Dizziness.
4. Weakness.
5. Sweating.
6. Hunger.
7. Irritability or moodiness.
8. Headache.
9. Blurry or double vision.
10. Pounding heartbeat.

11. Confusion.

    If left untreated, hypoglycaemia can lead to seizures and loss of consciousness.

    If you think that your blood sugar may be dipping too low, check your blood sugar level. Then eat or drink something that will raise your blood sugar level quickly for example, candy, sugar or glucose.

    If you experience symptoms of low blood sugar but can't check your blood sugar level right away, treat yourself as though you have hypoglycaemia. You should always carry glucose with you in your bag. It's also a good idea to wear a bracelet that identifies you as someone who has diabetes.

    Check your blood sugar level again 15-20 minutes later. If it's still too low, eat or drink something sugary. When you feel better, be sure to eat meals and snacks as usual. It is important that your family members also know your status and warning signs as they might be the ones offering you help in case of an emergency. Remind them to look for these red flags:

    i. Confusion.
    ii. Lack of coordination.
    iii. Strange behaviour.

Dental Health and Diabetes

Good dental health is important for your total well being.

1. To help prevent tooth decay and gum disease, guard your oral health by practicing proper brushing and flossing. Also, see your dentist regularly. Ask your dentist which type of brush will clean your teeth more effectively.

2. Flossing is the best way to remove food and plaque from between the teeth, an area the toothbrush cannot reach. Mouthwashes are generally used to temporarily freshen bad breath. Some mouthwashes may help reduce plaque levels. Fluoride mouthwashes also help protect the teeth against decay.

3. Prevent decay through nutrition. Decay occurs only when the inside of the mouth is acidic. This happens when you eat starchy or sugary foods (carbohydrates). You can help prevent decay by avoiding highly sugary or sticky foods, or brushing your teeth right after you eat these foods. Rinsing with water after you eat or drink sugar-containing foods can also help reduce the amount of acid and help wash away food plaque from the teeth which all promote good total well being.

Your best bet is to adopt a healthy diet – high in fruits, vegetables and whole grains.

How to Avoid Diabetic Complications

1. Make healthy eating and physical activity a part of your daily routine. Maintain a healthy weight. Monitor your blood sugar level and follow your doctor's instructions for keeping your blood sugar level within your target range.

2. Schedule yearly physicals and regular eye exams. During the physical, your doctor will look for any diabetes-related complication including signs of kidney damage, nerve damage and heart disease. The doctor will also screen for other medical problems. Your eye care specialist will check for signs of retinal damage, cataract and glaucoma.

3. Keep your vaccines up-to-date.

i. Flu Vaccine: A yearly flu vaccine can help you stay healthy during flu season, as well as prevent serious complications from the flu.
   ii. Pneumonia Vaccine: If you have diabetic complications or you are age is 65 or older, you may need a 5 year booster shot.
   iii. Other Vaccines: Stay up-to-date with your tetanus shot and it's 10 year boosters. Ask your doctor about the hepatitis B vaccine also.
4. Take care of your teeth. Diabetes may leave you prone to gum infections. Brush your teeth at least twice a day, floss your teeth once a day and schedule dental exams at least twice a year. Consult your dentist right away if your gums bleed or look red or swollen.
5. Pay attention to your feet. High blood sugar can damage the nerves in your feet and reduce blood flow to your feet. Left untreated, cuts and blisters can become serious infections. To prevent foot problems:
   i. Wash your feet daily in luke warm water.
   ii. Dry your feet gently, especially between the toes.
   iii. Moisturise your feet and ankles with a lotion.
   iv. Check your feet every day for blisters, cuts, sores, redness, or swelling.
   v. Consult your doctor if you have a sore or other foot problem that does not start to heal within a few days.
6. Keep your blood pressure and cholesterol under control.
7. Don't smoke.
8. Avoid alcohol.

Chapter 15

Raised Cholesterol Level (Hypercholesterolaemia)

High cholesterol levels (hypercholesterolaemia), is more commonly known as a reason for blockage of arteries. But what very few of us know is that cholesterol is found in every cell in our body and is essential for life. Cholesterol is used by our body to build healthy cells, as well as some vital hormones.

Abnormally high cholesterol levels (hypercholesterolaemia), or, more correctly, higher concentrations of LDL and lower concentrations of functional HDL are strongly associated with cardiovascular disease because these promote atheroma development in arteries (atherosclerosis). This disease process leads to myocardial infarction (heart attack), stroke and peripheral vascular disease. When you see your lipid profile report you come across terms like LDL and HDL but what do they mean? LDL particles are often termed **'bad cholesterol'** because they have been linked to atheroma formation. On the other hand, high concentrations of functional HDL, which can remove cholesterol from cells and atheroma, offer protection and are sometimes referred to colloquially as **'good cholesterol'**. High cholesterol (hypercholesterolaemia) is largely preventable and treatable. A healthy diet, regular exercise and sometimes medication can go a long way towards reducing high cholesterol although the balance between various components is genetically determined.

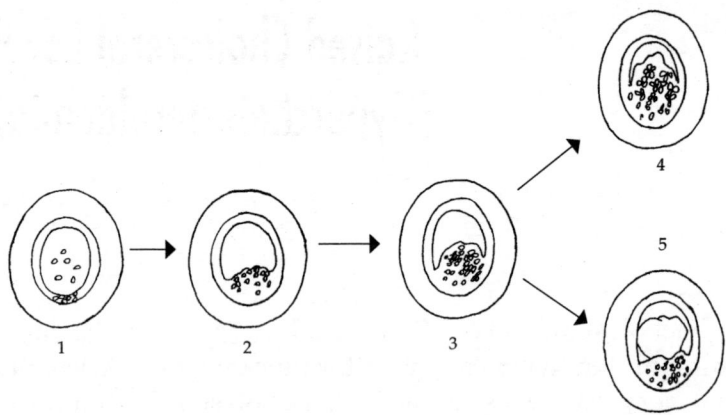

Fig. 15.1: The steps in plaque formation and growth. (1) cholesterol particles infiltrate the wall of the artery at the site of the damaged inner lining of the artery; (2) a plaque develops in the artery; (3) as more cholesterol and other materials are incorporated into the plaque, the plaque grows; (4) the plaque may continue to grow, blocking blood flow through the artery or (5) the plaque may 'rupture' and a blood clots may form, completely blocking blood flow through the artery.

Risk Factors

You're more likely to have high cholesterol that can lead to heart disease if you have any of these risk factors:

1. **Smoking:** Cigarette smoking damages the walls of your blood vessels, making them likely to accumulate fatty deposits. Smoking may also lower your level of HDL, or 'good', cholesterol.

2. **Obesity:** Having a body mass index (BMI) of 30 or greater puts you at a risk of high cholesterol.

3. **Poor Diet:** Foods that are high in cholesterol, such as red meat and full-fat dairy products, will increase your total cholesterol. Eating saturated fats, found in animal products and trans fats, found in some commercially baked cookies and cakes, also can raise your numbers.
4. **Lack of Exercise:** Exercise helps boost your body's HDL 'good' cholesterol while lowering your LDL 'bad' cholesterol.
5. **High Blood Pressure:** Increased pressure on your artery walls damages your arteries, which can speed the accumulation of fatty deposits.
6. **Diabetes:** High blood sugar contributes to higher LDL cholesterol and lower HDL cholesterol. High blood sugar also damages the lining of your arteries.
7. **Family History of Heart Disease:** If a parent or sibling developed heart disease before the age of 55, high cholesterol levels place you at a greater than average risk of developing heart disease.

Symptoms

High cholesterol has no symptoms. A blood test is the only way to detect high cholesterol. However, if the arteries that supply your heart with blood (coronary arteries) are affected, you may have chest pain (angina) and other symptoms of coronary artery disease.

If plaques tear or rupture, a blood clot may form at the plaque-rupture site blocking the flow of blood or breaking free and plugging an artery downstream. If blood flow to a part of your heart stops, you'll have a heart attack. If blood flow to a part of your brain stops, a stroke occurs.

A blood test to check cholesterol levels—called a **lipid profile** reports:

1. Total cholesterol.
2. LDL cholesterol.
3. HDL cholesterol.
4. Triglycerides—a type of fat in the blood.

For the most accurate measurements, do not eat or drink anything (other than water) for 12 hours before the blood sample is taken. The total blood cholesterol level should be: < 200 mg/dL which is considered to be normal cholesterol. It is recommended by the American Heart Association to test cholesterol every 5 years for people aged 20 years or older. It is recommended to have cholesterol tested more frequently than 5 years if a person has a total cholesterol of 200 mg/dL or more, a woman over the age of 45 years has HDL (good) cholesterol less than 40 mg/dL, or other risk factors for heart disease and stroke.

Control of Cholesterol Level

Cholesterol Absorption Inhibitors

1. **Statins:** Among the most commonly prescribed medications for lowering cholesterol—block a substance your liver needs to make cholesterol. This depletes cholesterol in your liver cells, which causes your liver to remove cholesterol from your blood.

2. **Bile-acid-binding Resins:** Liver uses cholesterol to make bile acids, a substance needed for digestion. This prompts the liver to use excess cholesterol to make more bile acids, which reduce the level of cholesterol in your blood.

Diet

Eat heart-healthy foods. What you eat has a direct impact on your cholesterol level. In fact, researchers say a diet rich in fibre and other cholesterol-lowering foods may help lower cholesterol as much as statin medication for some people.

1. **Choose Healthier Fats:** Get no more than 10 per cent of your daily calories from saturated fat. Monounsaturated fat—found in olive, peanut and canola oils—is a healthier option. Almonds and walnuts are other sources of healthy fats.

2. **Eliminate Trans Fats:** Trans fats, which are often found in margarines and commercially baked cookies, crackers and snack cakes, are particularly bad for your cholesterol levels. Not only do trans fats increase your total LDL 'bad' cholesterol, but they also lower your HDL 'good' cholesterol.

3. **Limit Your Dietary Cholesterol:** Avoiding animal products may decrease the cholesterol levels in the body. Those wishing to reduce their cholesterol through a change in diet should aim to consume less than 7 per cent of their daily calories from saturated fat and less than 200 mg of cholesterol per day. The most concentrated sources of cholesterol include organ meats, egg yolks and whole milk products. Use lean cuts of meat, egg substitutes and skimmed milk instead.

4. **Select Whole Grains:** Various nutrients found in whole grains promote heart health. Choose whole grain breads, whole wheat pasta, whole wheat flour and brown rice. Oatmeal and oat bran are other good choices.

5. **Stock Up on Fruits and Vegetables:** Fruits and vegetables are rich in dietary fibre, which can help lower cholesterol. Snack on seasonal fruits. Experiment with veggie-based casseroles, soups and stir-fries.

6. **Eat fish:** Some types of fish such as cod, tuna and halibut, have less total fat, saturated fat and cholesterol than meat and poultry. Salmon, mackerel and hering are rich in omega-3 fatty acids, which help promote heart health.

Avoid Alcohol

In some studies, moderate use of alcohol has been linked with higher levels of HDL cholesterol—but the benefits aren't strong enough to recommend alcohol for anyone who does not drink already. If you choose to drink, do so in moderation. This means no more than one drink a day for women and one to two drinks a day for men.

Exercise Regularly

Regular exercise can help improve your cholesterol levels. Work up to 30-60 minutes of exercise a day. And, you do not need to get all 30-60 minutes in one exercise session.

Lose Excess Weight

Excess weight contributes to high cholesterol. Losing even 5 to 10 pounds of excess weight can help lower total cholesterol levels.

Do not Smoke

If you smoke, stop. Quitting can improve your HDL cholesterol level.

Chapter 16

Obesity

According to an old saying, 'Middle age is when your age starts to show around your middle'. As one ages, the requirement of calories goes down. Also the basal metabolic rate, an entity which determines how well we burn our calories, become sluggish. Along with that if the amount of physical activity also decreases with age, or due to coexisting health problems like osteoarthritis and back pain then there are higher chances of accumulating fat. In middle-aged women, genetic factors remain the strongest influence on the amount and distribution of body fat. At the time of menopause, probably it is the oestrogen deficiency which is responsible for distribution of fat around the middle.

According to a survey of 2,000 women carried out in the UK, many women who are in their forties hate their bodies and many are developing eating disorders because of this. Infact, a significant number have had cosmetic surgery. As per some glaring facts revealed by this survey about women in their forties, most find losing weight much harder after 40, 58 per cent have disordered eating patterns and 70 per cent have made serious attempts to diet during the last 12 months. Most hate their middle, hips, thighs and upper arms. Over 30 per cent are regularly on one diet or another. Over 30 per cent take slimming pills or laxatives. Over half have had cosmetic surgery or would consider it. A vast majority of women put their weight gain down to getting older, having babies and menopause.

Obesity is a condition in which excess body fat has accumulated to an extent that health may be negatively affected. Obesity is commonly defined as a body mass index (BMI) of 30 kg/m^2 or higher. Waist hip ratio is also used to assess body fat.

Body Fat Percentage

Body fat percentage is total body fat expressed as a percentage of total body weight. It is generally agreed that men with more than 25 per cent body fat and women with more than 33 per cent body fat are obese. Body fat percentage can be estimated from a person's BMI.

It recognises that a person's percentage body fat increases as they age even if their weight remains constant.

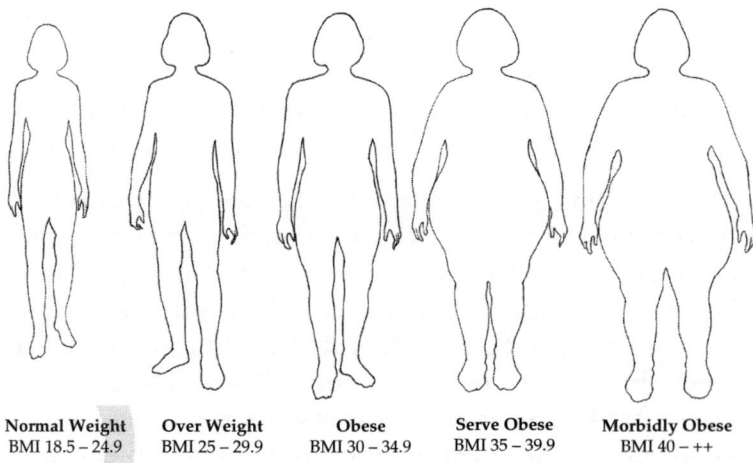

Normal Weight BMI 18.5 – 24.9   **Over Weight** BMI 25 – 29.9   **Obese** BMI 30 – 34.9   **Serve Obese** BMI 35 – 39.9   **Morbidly Obese** BMI 40 – ++

Fig. 16.1: A person's percentage body fat

Body mass index or BMI is a simple and widely used method for estimating body fat mass. BMI is an accurate reflection of body fat percentage in a majority of the adult population.

BMI	Classification
< 18.5	Underweight
18.5–24.9	Normal weight
25.0–29.9	Overweight
30.0–34.9	Class I obesity
35.0–39.9	Class II obesity
> 40.0	Class III obesity

BMI is calculated by dividing the subject's mass by the square of his or her height, typically expressed either in metric or US 'Customary' units:

Metric: BMI = kilograms / meters^2

US/Customary and imperial: BMI = lb * 703 / in^2

Where 'lb' is the subject's weight in pounds and 'in' is the subject's height in inches.

As Asian populations develop negative health consequences at a lower BMI than Caucasians, some nations have redefined obesity. The Japanese have defined obesity as any BMI greater than 25 while China uses a BMI of greater than 28.

The skin fold test, in which a pinch of skin is precisely measured to determine the thickness of the subcutaneous fat layer has been used in the past but it has its limitations.

Waist Circumference and Waist–Hip Ratio

The waist circumference (>102 cm in men and >88 cm in women) and the waist–hip ratio (the circumference of the waist divided by that of the hips of >0.9 for men and >0.85 for women) are both used as measures of central obesity.

Effects on Health

Excessive body weight is associated with various diseases, particularly cardiovascular diseases, diabetes mellitus type 2, obstructive sleep apnoea, certain types of cancer and osteoarthritis. As a result, obesity has been found to reduce life expectancy.

Management

The main treatment for obesity consists of dieting and physical exercise. Diet programmes may produce weight loss over the short term, but keeping this weight off can be a problem and often requires making exercise and a lower calorie diet a permanent part of a person's lifestyle. Success rates of long term weight loss maintenance are low and range from 2–20 per cent. In a more structured setting, however, 67 per cent of people who lost greater than 10 per cent of their body mass maintained or continued to lose weight one year later. An average maintained weight loss of more than 3 kg (6.6 lb) or 3 per cent of total body mass could be sustained for 5 years. There are significant benefits to weight loss. In a prospective study, intentional weight loss of any amount was associated with a 20 per cent reduction in all-cause mortality.

The most effective, but also most risky treatment for obesity is bariatric surgery. Due to its cost and risk of complications, researchers are fervently searching for new obesity treatments.

Dieting

Diets to promote weight loss are generally divided into four categories: Low fat, low carbohydrate, low calorie and very low calorie. A meta-analysis of six randomised controlled trials found no difference between the main diet types (low calorie, low carbohydrate and low fat), with a 2-4 kilograms (4.4–8.8 lb) weight loss in all studies. At 2 years, all diet methods resulted in similar weight loss irrespective of the macronutrients emphasized.

Low Fat Diets

Low fat diets involve reduction in the percentage of fat in one's diet. Calorie consumption is reduced but not purposely so. A meta-analysis of 16 trials of 2-12 months' duration found that low fat diets resulted in weight loss of 3.2 kg (7.1 lb) over eating as normal.

Low Carbohydrate Diets

Low carbohydrate diets such as Atkins and Protein Power are relatively high in fat and protein. They are very popular in the press but are not recommended by the American Heart Association. A review of 107 studies did not find that low carbohydrate diets cause weight loss, except when calorie intake was restricted. No adverse effects from low carbohydrate diets were detected.

Low Calorie Diets

Low calorie diets usually produce an energy deficit of 500–1,000 calories per day, which can result in a 0.5 kilograms (1.1 lb) weight loss per week. It includes the DASH diet. According to the National Institute of Health, these diets lowered the total body mass by 8 per cent over 3–12 months.

Very Low Calorie Diets

Very low calorie diets provide 200–800 kcal/day, maintaining protein intake but limiting calories from both fats and carbohydrates. They subject the body to starvation and produce an average weekly weight loss of 1.5–2.5 kilograms (3.3–5.5 lb). These diets are not recommended for general use as they are associated with adverse side effects such as loss of lean muscle mass, increased risks of gout and electrolyte imbalances. People attempting these diets must be monitored closely by a physician to prevent complications.

Exercise

With use, muscles consume energy derived from both fat and glycogen. Due to the large size of leg muscles, walking, running and cycling are the most effective means of exercise to reduce body fat. Exercise affects macronutrient balance. During moderate exercise, there is a shift to greater use of fat as a fuel.

It has been seen in trials that exercising alone led to limited weight loss. In combination with diet, however, it resulted in a 1 kilograms weight loss over dieting alone. A 1.5 kilograms (3.3 lb) loss was observed with a greater degree of exercise. Even though exercise, as carried out in the general population has only modest effects, very intense exercise can lead to substantial weight loss. High levels of physical activity seem to be necessary to maintain weight loss.

The city of Bogota, Colombia blocks off 113 kilometers (70 miles) of roads every Sunday and on holidays to make it easier for it's citizens to get exercise. These car-free zones are a part of an effort to combat chronic diseases, including obesity. 'Those who think they have no time for bodily exercise will sooner or later have to find time for illness'.

Medication

Only two anti-obesity medications are currently approved by the FDA for long term use. One is Orlistat (Xenical), which reduces intestinal fat absorption; the other is Sibutramine (Meridia), which acts on the brain to decrease appetite.

Weight loss with these drugs is modest; over the longer term, average weight loss on Orlistat is 2.9 kg (6.4 lb), Sibutramine is 4.2 kg (9.3 lb). There is however little data on how these drugs affect the longer term complications or outcomes of obesity.

Surgery

Bariatric surgery ('weight loss surgery') is only recommended for severely obese people who have failed to lose weight with dietary modification and drug therapy. Weight loss surgery relies on various principles; the most common approaches are reducing the volume of the stomach, producing an earlier sense of satiation (for example, by adjustable gastric banding) and reduce the length of bowel that food will be in contact with, directly reducing absorption (gastric bypass surgery). Band surgery is reversible, while bowel shortening operations are not. Complications from weight loss surgery are frequent and hence it should not be routinely advised.

Weight Loss Programmes

Weight loss programmes often promote lifestyle changes and diet modifications. This may involve eating smaller meals, by cutting down on certain types of food and making a conscious effort to exercise more. These programmes enable people to connect with a group of others who are attempting to lose weight in the hope that they will encourage and help each other out.

Fat Mass and Body Shape in Women of Menopausal Age

Risks of Increased Central Adiposity

Increased central adiposity in women is a greater predictor of heart disease, diabetes and death than generalised obesity. Central obesity is a part of the metabolic syndrome, with associated insulin resistance, dyslipidaemia and hypertension and glucose intolerance.

Effect of HRT on Obesity

Because weight gain is a feature of ageing, women taking hormone replacement therapy (HRT) may assume that any weight gain is a result of HRT. In reality, while weight gain is usual with time, it is not related to hormone administration: The Prospective Estrogen and Progestin Intervention (PEPI) study showed a similar mean increase in body weight in menopausal women receiving HRT and those receiving placebo. Data from the Massachusetts Women's Health Study also showed no relationship between weight gain and menopause, or HRT. However, it is notable that increases in weight were significantly related to cessation of smoking and discontinuation of exercise.

Many women have fought weight problems all their lives. Eating disorders and depression may be worsened by severe dieting; sensible eating habits for the rest of one's life should be encouraged rather than experimenting with different diets, then only one can say 'I am in shape, perfect shape!' and 'not I am in shape, round shape!' for the rest of our lives.

Chapter 17

Women and Heart Disease

In today's world, most deaths are attributed to non-communicable diseases (32 million) and just over half of these (16.7 million) are the result of cardiovascular diseases (CVD). More than one third of these deaths occur in middle aged adults. In developed countries, heart diseases and strokes are the first and the second leading causes of death for adult men and women. In developing countries also, CVD is emerging as a public health problem and the trend is rising. India falls in the group of high mortality countries and risk factors like tobacco use, high cholesterol and blood pressure are fast emerging.

As per the National Heart Lung and Blood Institute of the National Institutes of Health (NIH) 1 in 12 women aged 45 to 64 years has heart disease. 1 in 4 women over the age of 65 years has heart disease. Currently, 6.6 million women have heart disease.

A heart attack or myocardial infarction, occurs when blood flow to the heart is decreased on prolonged basis as a result of blockage in vessels supplying blood to the muscles of the heart. The blockage is due to a collection of fatty substances in the blood vessels which obstruct the flow of blood and oxygen to the heart.

Risk Factors for Heart Attack

There are two types of risk factors for heart attack, including the following:

Inherited or Genetic

1. Women with inherited hypertension—high blood pressure.
2. Women with inherited low levels of HDL (high density lipoprotein) or high levels of LDL (low density lipoprotein) blood cholesterol.
3. Women with a family history of heart disease (especially with onset before the age of 55 years).
4. Ageing women.
5. Women with type 1 diabetes.
6. Women, after the onset of menopause generally; men are at risk at an earlier age than women, but after the onset of menopause, women are equally at risk.

Acquired

1. Women with acquired hypertension—high blood pressure.
2. Women with acquired low levels of HDL (high density lipoprotein) or high levels of LDL (low density lipoprotein) blood cholesterol.
3. Cigarette smokers.
4. Women who are under a lot of stress.
5. Women who lead a sedentary lifestyle.
6. Women who are overweight by 30 per cent or more.

Warning Signs of Heart Attack

The following are the most common symptoms of a heart attack. However, each individual may experience symptoms differently. Symptoms may include:

1. Severe pressure, fullness, squeezing pain and/or discomfort in the center of the chest that lasts for more than a few minutes.

2. Pain or discomfort that spreads to the shoulders, neck, arms or jaw.

3. Chest pain that increases in intensity.

4. Chest pain that is not relieved by rest or by taking cardiac prescription medication.

5. Chest pain that occurs with any/all of the following (additional) symptoms:

    i. Sweating, cool clammy skin and/or paleness.

    ii. Shortness of breath.

    iii. Nausea or vomiting.

    iv. Dizziness or fainting.

    v. Unexplained weakness or fatigue.

    vi. Rapid or irregular pulse.

Although chest pain is the key warning sign of a heart attack, it may be confused with indigestion, pleurisy, pneumonia or other disorders.

The symptoms of a heart attack may resemble other medical conditions or problems. Always consult your physician for a diagnosis.

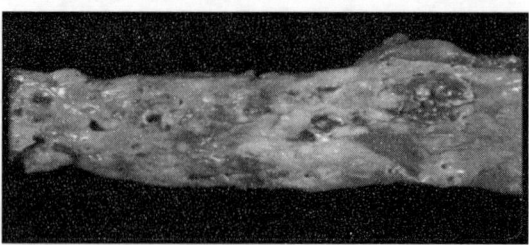

Fig. 17.1: Fat deposition

What Makes Women Different?

1. Chest pains in women are often attributed to causes other than coronary heart disease.

2. Both women and men may suffer 'classic' symptoms for a heart attack involving pain in the chest that spreads to the shoulders, neck, or arms.

3. Women sometimes have atypical chest pain or abdominal pain and nausea, difficulty in breathing or fatigue as the early symptoms of a heart attack. These atypical symptoms make it more difficult to diagnose.

4. Women tend to have heart attacks later in life than men. Advanced age may explain the greater mortality rate of women from heart attacks.

5. Some diagnostic tests, such as the exercise stress test, may not be as accurate in women. This may delay detection of the disease until it is advanced.

6. Single vessel heart disease is more common in women and is not as readily picked up on a routine stress test (ECG).

Diagnosis

The following are just a few of the diagnostic tests that have been used/are being used to further understand and identify cardiovascular diseases:

Electrocardiogram (ECG or EKG)

A test that records the electrical activity of the heart, shows abnormal rhythms (arrhythmias) and detects heart muscle damage.

Stress Test

(Usually with ECG; also called treadmill or exercise ECG). A test that is given while a patient walks on a treadmill or pedals a stationary bike to monitor the heart during exercise. Breathing and blood pressure rates are also monitored. A stress test may be used to detect coronary artery disease, and/or to determine safe levels of exercise following a heart attack or heart surgery.

Echocardiogram (ECHO)

A non-invasive test that uses sound waves to produce a study of the motion of the heart's chambers and valves. The echo sound waves create an image on the monitor as an ultrasound transducer is passed over the heart.

Transesophageal Echocardiogram (TEE)

A test in which a small transducer is passed down the esophagus to provide a clearer image of the heart structure.

Coronary Arteriogram (Angiogram)

With this procedure, x-rays are taken after a contrast agent is injected into an artery to locate the narrowing, occlusions and other abnormalities of specific arteries.

Positron Emission Tomography (PET) Scan

A nuclear scan that gives information about the flow of blood through the coronary arteries to the heart muscle.

PET F-18 FDG (Fluorodeoxyglucose) Scan

A glucose scan sometimes done immediately after the PET scan to determine if the heart muscle has any permanent damage.

Thallium Scans or Myocardial Perfusion Scans

MUGA Scans/Radionuclide Angiography (RNA) Scan

Holter Monitor

A small, portable, battery-powered ECG machine is worn by a patient to record heartbeats on tape over a period of 24–48 hours, during normal activities. At the end of the time period, the monitor is returned to the physician's office so the tape can be read and evaluated.

Tilt Table Test

It is a test performed while the patient is connected to an ECG and blood pressure monitors and strapped to a table that tilts in different directions. This test is done to determine if the patient is prone to sudden drops in blood pressure or slow pulse rates.

Electrophysiology Study

A test in which insulated electric catheters are placed inside the heart to study the heart`s electrical system

Cardiac Catheterization

It is a test in which a small catheter (hollow tube) is guided through a vein or artery into the heart. An iodine compound (a colourless, liquid "dye") is given through the catheter and moving X-ray pictures are made as the dye travels through the heart. This comprehensive test narrowing in the arteries, outside heart size, inside chamber size, pumping ability of the heart, ability of the valves to open and close, as well as a measurement of the pressures within the heart.

Treatment

The goal of treatment for a heart attack is to relieve pain, preserve the heart muscle function and prevent death.

Treatment in the emergency department may include:

1. Intravenous therapy.
2. Continuous monitoring of the heart and vital signs.
3. Oxygen therapy (to improve oxygenation to the damaged heart muscle).
4. Pain medication (by decreasing pain, the workload of the heart decreases, thus the oxygen demand of the heart decreases).
5. Cardiac medication (to promote blood flow to the heart, prevent blood clotting, improve the blood supply, prevent arrhythmias and decrease heart rate and blood pressure).
6. Thrombolytic therapy (intravenous infusion of a medication which dissolves the blockage, thus restoring blood flow).

Once the condition has been diagnosed and the patient stabilised, additional procedures to restore coronary blood flow may be utilised, including the following:

Coronary Angioplasty

With this procedure, a catheter is used to create a larger opening in the vessel to increase blood flow. Although angioplasty is performed in other blood vessels, percutaneous transluminal coronary angioplasty (PTCA) refers to angioplasty in the coronary arteries to permit more blood flow into the heart. There are several types of PTCA procedures, including the following:

1. **Balloon Angioplasty:** A small balloon is inflated inside the blocked artery to open the blocked area.
2. **Atherectomy:** The blocked area inside the artery is 'shaved' away by a tiny device on the end of a catheter.
3. **Laser Angioplasty:** A laser is used to 'vaporize' the blockage in the artery.
4. **Coronary Artery Stent:** A tiny coil is expanded inside the blocked artery to open the blocked area and is left in place to keep the artery open.

Coronary Artery Bypass

Coronary artery bypass is a surgical procedure in which small portions of veins or arteries are taken from one part of the body and transplanted into the heart to bypass clogged coronary arteries in the heart.

Managing your risks for a heart attack begins with finding the high risk factors which are applicable to you. Also knowing which factors are modifiable and which non-modifiable helps. Consult your physician and try and control them. Remember heart attack is preventable.

If you have a person with a known history of heart disease, the phone number of the physician along with ambulance contact numbers should be kept handy.

How to perform CPR (Cardio-pulmonary Resuscitation)

Conventional CPR is performed by qualified medical practitioners; however, a layman can also carry out CPR for maintaining circulation and breathing. It involves clearing the airway, mouth-to-mouth rescue breathing along with chest compression.

1. Call for help.

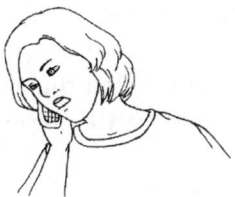

Fig. 17.2: Calling for help

2. Before doing CPR, put the person on his/her back and try to wake him/her up. Check whether the person is conscious or unconscious. If it is confirmed that he/she is in an unconscious state, then only one can proceed for CPR. The first step in performing CPR is to open the airway of the person. To achieve this, put your palm on the forehead and carefully tilt the head back. Gently lift the chin forward with your other hand and try to feel the person's breath. Also look if there is any chest movement. If the person is not breathing properly, pinch the nostrils and seal his/her mouth with yours. Now, you can give a mouth-to-mouth breathing for one second. Check for any rise of the chest. If yes, let the chest fall and repeat the procedure twice.

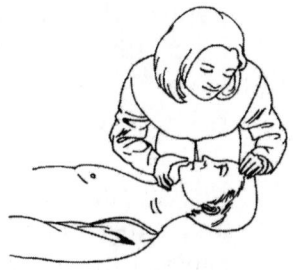

Fig. 17.3: Mouth-to-mouth breathing

In case, the chest does not rise, repeat the step of clearing the airway (head-tilt, chin-rise) position and do mouth-to-mouth breathing again. If the mouth is injured, one can give mouth-to-nose breathing.

3. Now, proceed with chest compressions in order to restore the blood circulation of the person. For this, kneel at the side of the person and place the heel of your hand in the middle of the chest (between the nipples). You have to put your other hand on top of the hand placed on the chest. Make sure your elbows are straight and the shoulders are directly above the hand.

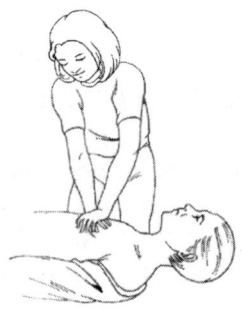

Fig. 17.4: Chest compression

Gently compress the chest of the victim to about 5 cms (2 inches). While giving chest compression, push hard and fast at a rate of about 2 per second. Repeat the compression 30 times and after that, open the airway as mentioned in the first step. Give 2 rescue breaths and check if the chest rises. This is the completion of the first cycle.

Repeat the steps, about 5 cycles of 30 compressions and 2 rescue breaths that is, for about 2 minutes and check if the person starts breathing or not. In case the person is not breathing, repeat the procedure again until help arrives.

Chapter 18

Osteoporosis

Osteoporosis literally means porous bones. It is a disease of the bones in which the bone mineral density (BMD) is reduced. Osteoporotic bones are more at risk of fracture. It is a silent killer as there are no symptoms of the disease and most people consult the doctor too late in time.

On an average, 1 in 2 women over 50 years of age will have an osteoporosis-related fracture in their lifetime. But in India, the incidence is higher–1 in 3-4 women get osteoporosis before the age of 50. Osteoporosis fractures occur 10-20 years earlier in Indians compared to people in western countries. For women there are dual concerns as they are not able to perform well at work and their domestic life also suffers

Osteoporosis, although asymptomatic for most part leads to falls and fractures making it a serious concern. Porous bones require lesser pressure and strain to fracture as compared to normal healthy bones. There is always a constant remodelling of bones, where bone formation is performed by the osteoblast cells, whereas bone resorption is accomplished by osteoclast osteoclast cells.

Bone remodelling is heavily influenced by nutritional and hormonal factors. Calcium and vitamin D, parathyroid hormone, glucorticoid hormones, calcitonin, oestrogen, testosterone and follicle stimulating hormone (FSH) all affect the bone mineral density. `Resorption', the process of releasing calcium from bones into the blood, results in the breakdown of bones. By another process called `formation', the bones get rebuilt. Together, the two processes constitute bone remodelling.

Signs and Symptoms

Typical fragility fractures occur in the vertebral column, hip and wrist. Collapse of a vertebra (**'compression fracture'**) can cause numbness in the right second toe or one or a combination of the following: Acute onset of back pain; a hunched forward or bent stature; loss of height; limited mobility and possibly disability. Fractures of the long bones acutely impair mobility and may require surgery. Hip fracture, in particular, usually requires prompt surgery, as

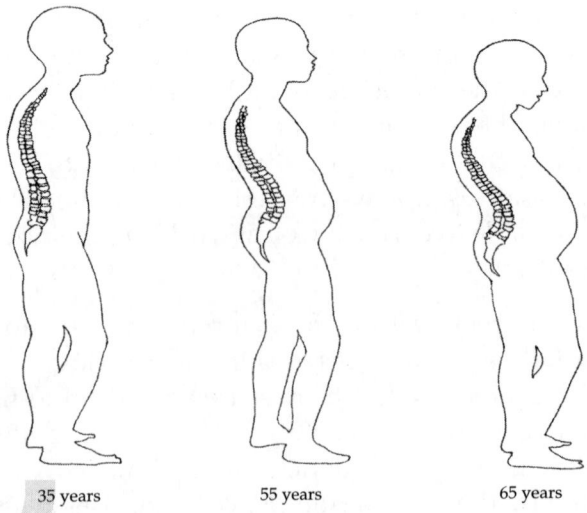

35 years   55 years   65 years

Fig. 18.1: Showing changes in vertebral column with age

there are serious risks associated with a hip fracture, such as deep vein thrombosis and a pulmonary embolism.

Risk Factors

Risk factors for osteoporotic fracture can be split between modifiable and non-modifiable factors.

Non-modifiable Risk Factors

1. **Sex:** Your chances of developing osteoporosis are greater if you are a woman. Women have lower peak bone mass and smaller bones than men. They also lose bone more rapidly than men in middle age because of the dramatic reduction in oestrogen levels that occurs with menopause.
2. **Age:** The older you are, the greater your risk of osteoporosis. Bone loss builds up over time and your bones become weaker as you age.
3. **Body Size:** Slender, thin-boned and taller women are at greater risk.
4. **Race:** Caucasian (white) and Asian women are at highest risk. African-American and Hispanic women have a lower but significant risk. Among men, Caucasians are at a higher risk than others. These differences in risk can be explained in part, though not entirely, by differences in peak bone mass among these groups.
5. **Family History:** Susceptibility to osteoporosis and fractures appears to be, in part, hereditary.
6. **History of Fracture** as an adult.
7. **Oestrogen Deficiency:** Deficiency following menopause is correlated with a rapid reduction in BMD.

Modifiable Risk Factors

1. **Sex Hormone Deficiencies:** The most common manifestation of oestrogen deficiency in premenopausal women is amenorrhoea—the abnormal absence of menstrual periods. Missed or irregular periods can be caused by various factors, including hormonal disorders as well as extreme levels of physical activity combined with restricted calorie intake. For example, in female athletes.

2. **Diet:** From childhood to old age, a diet low in calcium and vitamin D can increase your risk of osteoporosis and fractures. Excessive dieting or inadequate caloric intake can also be bad for bone health. People who are very thin and do not have much body fat to cushion falls have an increased risk of fracture too.

3. **Certain Medical Conditions:** In addition to sex hormone problems and eating disorders, other medical conditions—including a variety of genetic, endocrine, gastrointestinal, blood and rheumatic disorders and anorexia nervosa are associated with an increased risk for osteoporosis. Late onset of puberty and early menopause reduce lifetime oestrogen exposure in women and also increase the risk of osteoporosis.

4. **Medications:** Long term use of certain medications, including glucocorticoids and some anti-convulsants, leads to bone loss and increased risk of osteoporosis. Other drugs that may lead to bone loss include anti-clotting drugs, such as heparin; drugs that suppress the immune system, such as cyclosporine; and drugs used to treat prostate cancer.

5. **Sedentary Lifestyle:** An inactive lifestyle or extended bed rest also make a person prone to osteoporosis.

6. **Excessive Use of Alcohol:** Chronic heavy drinking is a significant risk factor for osteoporosis.
7. **Smoking.**

Diagnosis

1. **Bone Densitometry :** It is a radiological test which can diagnose osteoporosis early enough and treat it. This procedure does not require hospital admission and is painless. Depending on the type of machine, you may be asked to lie down or put your ankle in a device. Most machines use X-rays. A densitometry machine calculates the bone density and prepares a chart comparing the real values with those considered to be normal. If the bone density is less, it indicates osteoporosis and a physician by looking at it makes a diagnosis. More the density, stronger the bone.

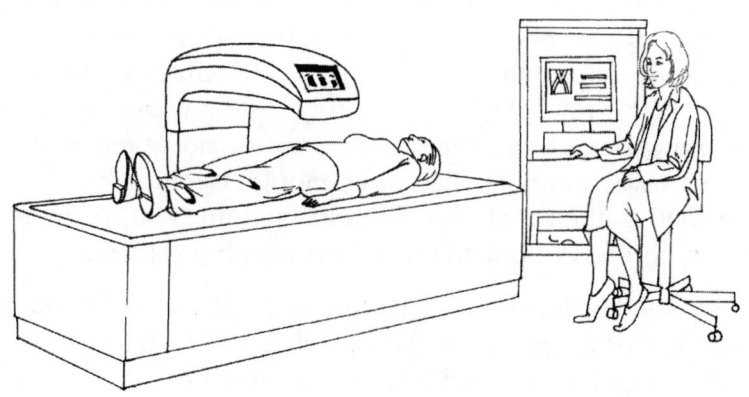

Fig. 18.2: Radiological test to diagnose osteoporosis

2. **Urine NTx:** The rate of bone turnover, on the other hand, can be measured with urine NTx, a by-product of bone cartilage breakdown. Urine NTx greater than 40 may indicate osteoporosis.

Today, many cases of osteoporosis in developed countries are diagnosed before symptoms develop. This is due to widespread screening for osteoporosis using the **DXA scan**. With treatment, bone mineral density increases and fracture risk decreases.

Treatment

Two things are important while starting the treatment: One is prevention of fracture in osteoporotic individuals and the other is to correct the underlying cause of osteoporosis.

Nutrition

A healthy, balanced diet that includes plenty of fruits and vegetables; enough calories; and adequate calcium, vitamin D and vitamin K is essential for minimising bone loss and maintaining overall health. Calcium and vitamin D are especially important for bone health. Calcium is the most important nutrient for preventing osteoporosis and for reaching peak bone mass. For healthy post-menopausal women who are not consuming enough calcium (1,200 mg per day) in their diet, calcium and vitamin D supplements help to preserve bone mass and prevent hip fracture.

Good sources of calcium include low fat dairy products; dark green leafy vegetables, including broccoli and turnip greens; sardines and salmon with bones; soy beans, tofu and other soy products; and calcium fortified foods such as orange juice, cereals and breads. If there is not enough calcium in your diet, calcium supplements can be taken but the total intake should not exceed 2,500 mg as there is a risk of kidney stones.

Vitamin D

Although many people are able to obtain enough vitamin D naturally, vitamin D production decreases in the elderly, in people who are housebound or do not get enough sun and in some people with chronic neurological or gastrointestinal diseases. These individuals and others at risk for vitamin D deficiency may require vitamin D supplementation. The recommended daily intake of vitamin D is 200 international units (IU) for adults up to the age of 50 years; 400 IU for men and women aged 51 to 70; and 600 IU for people over 70 years. Consuming more than 2,000 IU of vitamin D per day (or 1,000 IU for infants) can cause serious health problems.

Lifestyle

In addition to a healthy diet, a healthy lifestyle is important for optimising bone health. You should avoid smoking and if you drink alcohol, do so in moderation (no more than one drink per day is a good general guideline). It is also important to recognise that some prescription medications can cause bone loss or increase your risk of falling and breaking a bone.

Exercise

Exercise is an important part of an osteoporosis treatment programmes. Physical activity is needed to build and maintain bones throughout adulthood and complete bed rest leads to serious bone loss. Evidence suggests that the most beneficial physical activities for bone health include strength training or resistance training.

Fall Prevention

Falls can also be caused by factors in your environment that create unsafe conditions. Some tips to help eliminate the environmental factors that lead to falls include:

1. Use a cane for added stability.
2. Wear shoes that give good support and have non-slip soles.
3. Be careful on highly polished floors and wet floors.
4. Keep rooms free of clutter, especially on floors.
5. Be sure staircases are well lit and that stairs have handrails.
6. Install grab bars on bathroom walls near tub, shower and toilet.
7. Use a rubber bath mat in the shower.
8. You can use a cordless phone so that you do not have to rush to answer the phone when it rings.
9. Edges of the carpets, rugs, floor mats should be well sealed.
10. Get a light fixed at the entrance of every door so that you can switch the light on before entering the room.
11. Get your vision and distant vision checked and corrected as it could be associated with falls.

Prevention

Smoking

Smoking is bad for your bones and for your heart and lungs. Women who smoke have lower levels of oestrogen compared to non-smokers and frequently go through menopause earlier.

Alcohol

People who drink heavily are more prone to bone loss and fractures because of poor nutrition and harmful effects on calcium balance and hormonal factors. Drinking too much also increases the risk of falling, which is likely to increase fracture risk.

Medications That Cause Bone Loss

The long term use of glucocorticoids can lead to a loss of bone density and fractures. Other forms of drug therapy that can cause bone loss include long term treatment with certain anti-seizure drugs, such as phenytoin (Dilantin) and barbiturates; some drugs used to treat endometriosis; excessive use of aluminum-containing antacids; certain cancer treatments; and excessive thyroid hormone. It is important to discuss the use of these drugs with your doctor and not to stop or alter your medication dose on your own.

Prevention Medications

Beside its effects on your bones, osteoporosis can change your life in many other ways. These include anxiety and depression, limitations in the ability to work and enjoy leisure activities, acute or chronic pain difficulties in performing the activities of daily life.

Exercise

Weight bearing exercise is of great importance for people suffering from osteoporosis because it helps build bone density and strength.

Thirty minutes of weight-bearing exercise such as walking or jogging, three times a week, has shown to increase bone mineral density and reduce the risk of falls by strengthening the major muscle groups in the legs and back.

Exercises for Osteoporosis

Exercise is an important part of an osteoporosis treatment programme.

Before You Start

Consult your doctor before starting any exercise programme for osteoporosis. You may need a bone density test and a fitness assessment first.

In the meantime, think about what kind of activities you enjoy most. If you choose an exercise you enjoy, you are more likely to stick with it over time.

Choosing the Right Form of Exercise

Three types of activities are often recommended for people with osteoporosis:

1. Strength training exercises, especially those for the back.
2. Weight-bearing aerobic activities.
3. Flexibility exercises.

Strength Training

Strength training includes the use of free weights, weight machines, resistance bands or water exercises to strengthen the muscles and bones in your arms and upper spine. Strength training can also work directly on your bones to slow mineral loss.

Osteoporosis can cause compression fractures in your spinal column. These fractures often lead to a stooped posture, increasing the pressure along the front of your spinal column and result in even more compression fractures. Exercises that gently stretch your upper back, strengthen the muscles between your shoulder blades and improve your posture can all help to reduce harmful stress on your bones and maintain bone density.

Weight-bearing Aerobic Activities

Weight-bearing aerobic activities involve doing aerobic exercise on your feet, with your bones supporting your weight. Examples include walking, dancing, low impact aerobics, elliptical training machines, stair climbing and gardening. These types of exercises work directly on the bones in your legs, hips and lower spine to slow mineral loss. They can also provide cardiovascular benefits, which boost heart and circulatory system health.

Swimming and water aerobics have many benefits, but they do not have the impact your bones need to slow mineral loss. However, these activities can be useful in cases of extreme osteoporosis, during rehabilitation following a fracture or for only increasing aerobic capacity.

Flexibility Exercises

Being able to move your joints through their full range of motion helps you maintain good balance and prevent muscle injury. Increased flexibility can also help improve your posture. When your joints are stiff, your abdominal and chest muscles become tight, pulling you forward and giving you a stooped posture.

Stretches are best performed after your muscles are warmed up—at the end of your exercise session, for example. They should be done gently and slowly, without bouncing. Avoid stretches that flex your spine or cause you to bend at the waist. These positions may put excessive stress on the bones in your spine (vertebrae), placing you at greater risk of a compression fracture.

Movements to Avoid

If you have osteoporosis, do not do the following types of exercises:

1. **High-Impact Exercises:** such as jumping, running or jogging. These activities increase compression in your spine and lower extremities and can lead to fractures in weakened bones. Avoid jerky, rapid movements in general. Choose exercises with slow, controlled movements.

2. **Exercises in Which You Bend Forward and Twist Your Waist:** Such as touching your toes, doing sit-ups or using a rowing machine. These movements also put pressure on the bones in your spine, increasing your risk of compression fractures. Other activities that may require you to bend or twist forcefully at the waist are golf, tennis, bowling and some yoga poses.

Exercise Tips

1. Even if you do not have osteoporosis, you should check with your health care provider before you start an exercise programme.

2. Remember to warm up before starting and cool down at the end of each exercise session.

3. For the best benefit to your bone health, combine several different weight-bearing exercises.

4. As you build strength, increase resistance or weights, rather than repetitions.

5. Remember to drink plenty of water whenever exercising.

6. Combine weight-bearing and resistance exercises with aerobic exercises to help improve your overall health.

7. Add more physical activity to your day; take the stairs instead of the elevator, park further way and walk to your co-worker's office rather than emailing.

Type of Exercises

Overhead Press

Stand or sit with spine in neutral alignment and feet hip-width apart. Start with elbows extended and weights level with top of your head.

Exhale as you press weights towards the ceiling, straightening your elbows.

Inhale as you lower weights to start position. Feel the workout in the top of your shoulders and upper arms. Don't stress or strain your neck.

Triceps Kick-back

With weight in right hand keep spine in a neutral position as you lean on a chair with the left hand. Left foot is kept forward and the knee is slightly bent; right leg is behind and straight.

Bring right upper arm next to your body and hold it still throughout the exercise.

Exhale as you straighten the elbow, extending the weight back behind you.

Inhale as you slowly bend the elbow. Feel work in the back of your upper arm and shoulder.

Bent-over Rows

Weight in right hand, keep spine in a neutral position as you lean on a chair with the left hand. Left foot is forward and knee is slightly bent; right leg is behind and straight.

Start with right arm straight and the weight pointing at the floor on a slight forward angle.

Exhale to draw weight to your side, bending elbow. Feel work in your shoulder blade and back of arm.

Inhale to slowly lower weight to start position.

Biceps Curl

Stand with feet hip-width apart, weights at your sides, palm facing forward.

Exhale as you bend elbows to draw weights towards your shoulders. Feel work in the front of your upper arm.

Keep upper arm and trunk still. Inhale to lower weights to start position

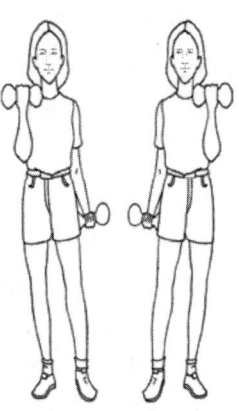

Fig. 18.3: Biceps curl

Do not stress or strain your neck. Even if you have limitations or are stuck in an office for most of the week, you can still experience the positive effects of this exercise. All you need to perform these chair exercises means exercises which can be done indoors by using a chair. is a little time, 15-20 minutes and maybe some privacy.

Chair Exercises

Chair exercises means exercises which can be done in doors by using a chair. The chair exercises are especially good for seniors with mobility problems, or persons suffering from back problems or cardiovascular disorders. It is also good for persons with balance problems.

These chair exercises can also be done by fit people as a change of pace or when the opportunity presents itself at work. **Warm up**, if at all possible. Whether you are doing these exercises due to limitations or doing chair exercises for seniors or office workers, try preceding routine with a warm up. Anything will do as long as your body temperature is raised a few degrees. A five minute walk would be sufficient. It would be even better if you could swing your arms. Stuck in an office, just march in place, stepping as high as you can.

Effects of exercise are improved after a warm up and negative effects of exercise, like soreness and injury may be reduced by warming up.

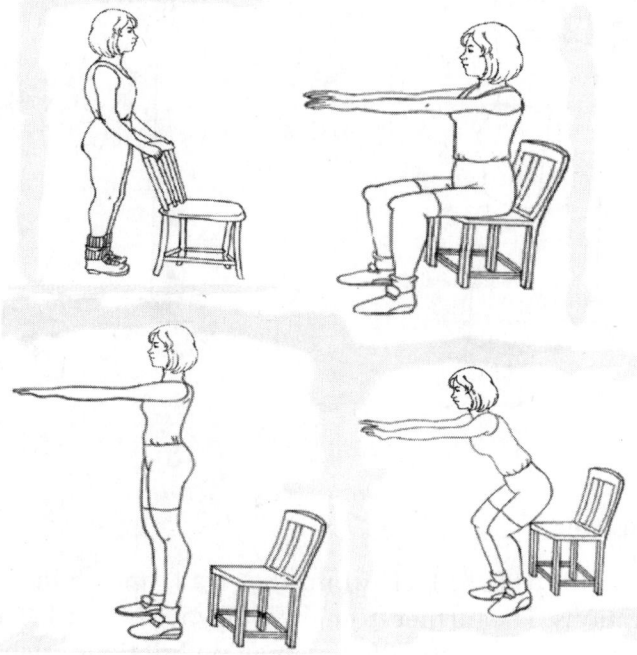

Fig. 18.4: Chair exercises

Squats

Squats will really help tone the large muscles of the legs.

Using a chair will help prevent certain errors that could lead to injury, like squatting too deeply. Squat as figures suggest not allowing knees to move in front of toes. I like to start from a sitting position, squatting up and immediately returning to sitting position.

1 to 3 sets of 5 - 50 repetitions (as per the stamina of the person).

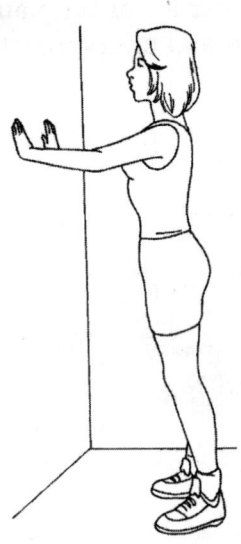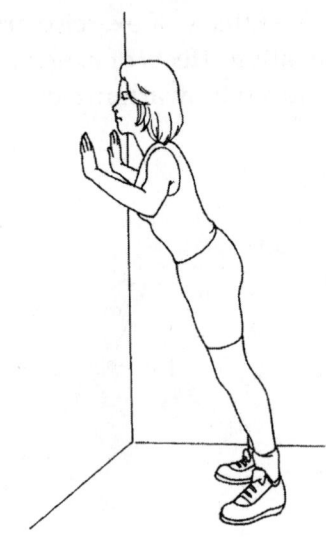

Fig. 18.5: Wall push ups

Wall Push Ups

Stand a few feet from the wall and follow the illustrations. The further from the wall you stand, the harder the movement. Eventually, you may do full floor push ups.

1 to 3 sets of 3 to 25 repetitions(as per the stamina of the person).

Heel Raises

This exercise tones your calf muscles.

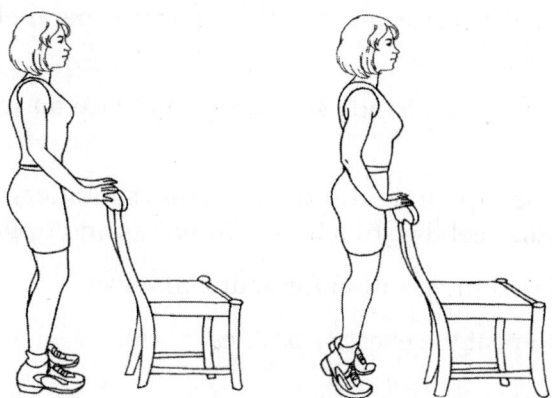

Fig. 18.6: Heel raises

Balance yourself behind a chair and raise your heels off the floor. The higher you go, the greater the effect. As you get better at this, you can hold weights for increased resistance. Better still, you can do heel raises on one leg.

1 to 2 sets of 5 to 50 repetitions (as per the stamina of the person).

Finger Exercise/Chair

This movement stretches your wrists and upper back.

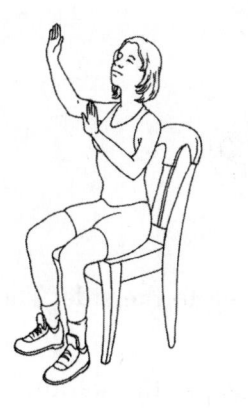 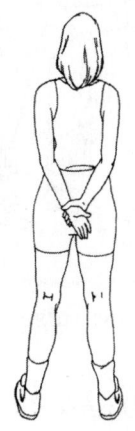 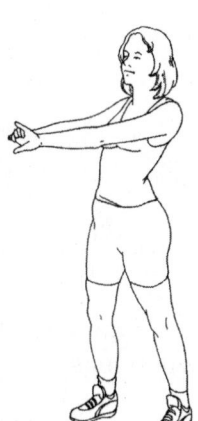

Fig. 18.7: Finger exercise

Raise your arms so that they're parallel to the ground.

Rotate your hands so your palms face an imaginary wall.

Stand up straight, but curl your shoulders forward. You should feel the stretch in your wrists and upper back.

Hold the position for about 10 seconds.

Repeat the exercise 3 times.

Side Hip Raise

Tones hips, thighs and butt. Also strengthens hip bones.

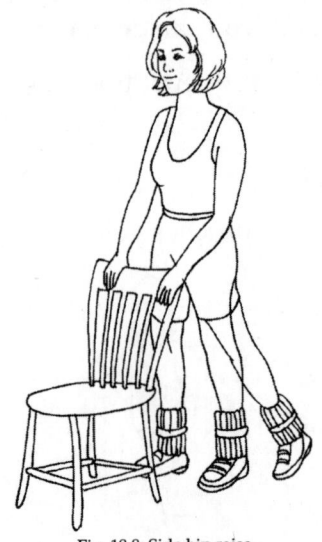

Fig. 18.8: Side hip raise

Stand as pictured and raise one leg to the side. Then switch legs.

1 to 2 sets of 8 of 20 repetitions (as per the stamina of the person).

Knee Extension

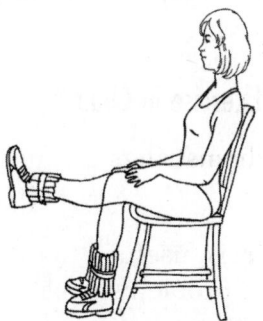

Fig. 18.9: Knee extension

Targets upper front thighs.

Sit comfortably and extend one knee until the entire leg is parallel to the floor. Switch legs.

You can add ankle weights for greater resistance.

1 to 2 sets of 5 to 40 repetitions (as per the stamina of the person).

Knee Curl

Strengthens the muscles of the upper back legs (hamstrings).

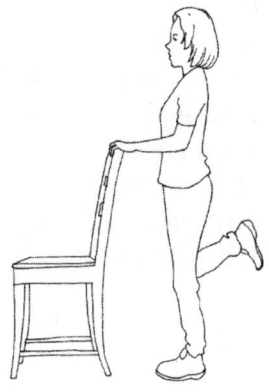

Fig. 18.10: Knee curl

1 to 2 sets of 5 to 40 repetitions (as per the stamina of the person).

Hamstring/Calf Stretch Exercise in Chair

Stretches the hamstrings and calves.

Using the chair is useful for persons with back problems or cardiovascular disorders.

1 to 2 sets of 5 to 30 repetitions (as per the stamina of the person).

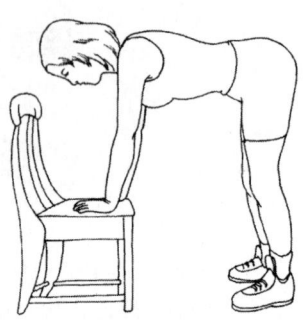

Fig. 18.11: Calf stretch exercise

Quadraceps Stretch Exercise/ Chair

Stretches the muscles on the front thighs.

1 - 2 sets, 5 - 30 seconds

Do this exercise in chair routine 3 – 5 times weekly for a few weeks.

Then start to expand your routine. Even if you are a senior or have limitations, you should be able to add walks, some light resistance exercises, an appropriate sport to round out your fitness routines and prevent burn out and boredom.

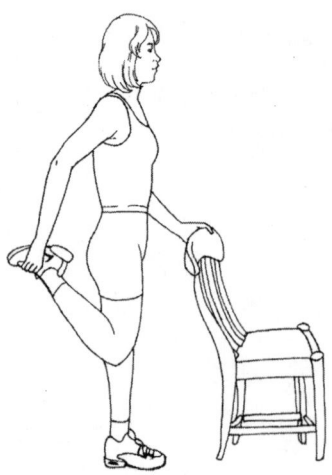

Fig. 18.12: Quadraceps stretch exercise

Chapter 19

Osteoarthritis

Osteoarthritis is a type of arthritis that is caused by the breakdown and eventual loss of the cartilage of one or more joints. Cartilage is a protein substance that serves as a 'cushion' between the bones of the joints. Osteoarthritis is also known as degenerative arthritis. Osteoarthritis occurs more frequently as we age. After the age of 55 years, it occurs more frequently in females. It affects millions of individuals all over the world.

Most cases of osteoarthritis have no known cause and are referred to as primary osteoarthritis. When the cause of the osteoarthritis is known, the condition is referred to as secondary osteoarthritis.

Causes

1. **Age:** Primary osteoarthritis is mostly related to aging. With aging, the water content of the cartilage increases and the protein make up of cartilage degenerates. Eventually, the cartilage begins to degenerate. Repetitive use of the worn our joints over the years

can irritate and inflame the cartilage, causing joint pain, swelling and limitation of joint mobility. Osteoarthritis commonly affects the hands, feet, spine and large weight-bearing joints, such as the hips and knees.

2. **Genetic:** Many members of the same family are affected.

3. **Other Medical Conditions:** Secondary osteoarthritis may be caused by obesity, repeated trauma or surgery to the joint structures, abnormal joints at birth (congenital abnormalities), gout, diabetes and other hormonal disorders. Obesity causes osteoarthritis by increasing the mechanical stress on the cartilage.

Symptoms

Osteoarthritis is a disease of the joints. It does not affect other organs of the body. The most common symptom of osteoarthritis is pain in the affected joint(s) after repetitive use. Joint pain is usually worse later in the day. There can be swelling, warmth and creaking of the affected joints. Pain and stiffness of the joints can also occur after long periods of inactivity, for example, sitting in one place during a journey. In severe osteoarthritis, complete loss of cartilage cushion causes friction between bones, resulting in pain at rest or pain with limited motion. Symptoms can also be intermittent. It is not unusual for patients with osteoarthritis of the finger joints of the hands and knees to have years of pain-free intervals between symptoms. Osteoarthritis of the knees is often associated with excess upper body weight, with obesity, or a history of repeated injury and/or joint surgery. Progressive cartilage degeneration of the knee joints can lead to outward curvature of the knees referred to as 'bow legs'.

Osteoarthritis

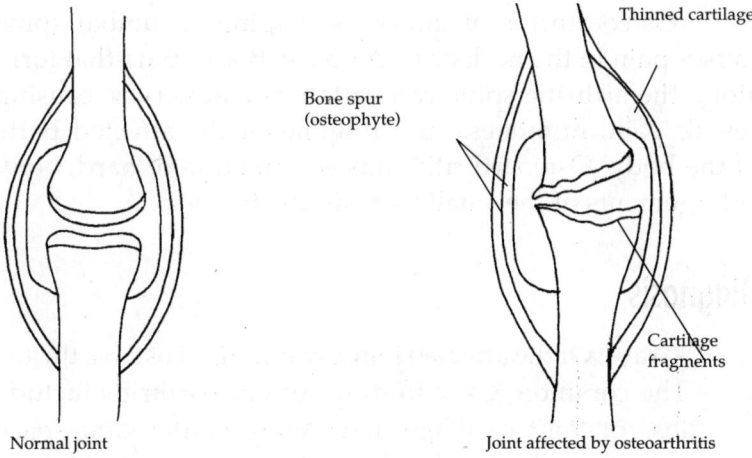

Fig. 19.1: Osteoarthritic joint

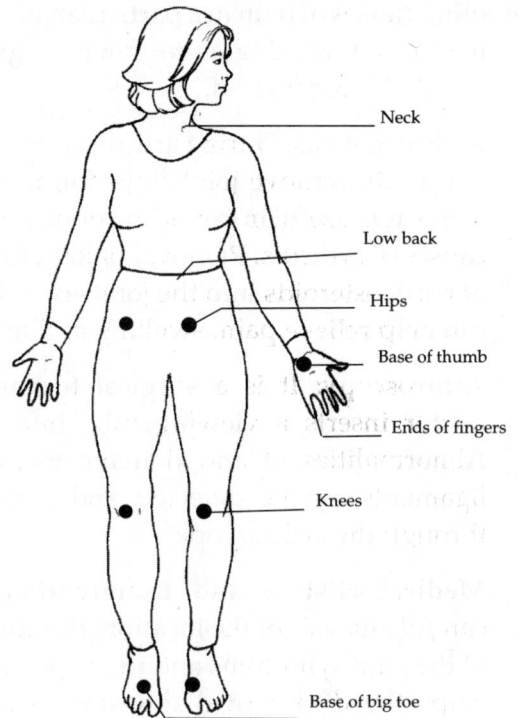

Fig. 19.2: The joints most often affected by osteoarthritis

Osteoarthritis of the cervical spine or lumbar spine causes pain in the neck or lower back. Bony spurs that form along the arthritic spine can irritate spinal nerves, causing severe pain, numbness and tingling of the affected parts of the body. Osteoarthritis causes formation of hard, bony enlargements of the small joints in the fingers.

Diagnosis

1. **X-rays:** Of the affected joints can suggest osteoarthritis. The common X-ray findings of osteoarthritis include loss of joint cartilage, narrowing of the joint space between adjacent bones and bone spur formation. Simple X-ray testing can be very helpful to exclude other causes of pain in a particular joint as well as assist in decision making as to when surgical intervention should be considered.

2. **Arthrocentesis:** During arthrocentesis, a sterile needle is used to remove joint fluid for analysis. Joint fluid analysis is useful in excluding gout, infection and other causes of arthritis. Removal of joint fluid and injection of corticosteroids into the joints during arthrocentesis can help relieve pain, swelling and inflammation.

3. **Arthroscopy:** It is a surgical technique whereby a doctor inserts a viewing tube into the joint space. Abnormalities of and damage to the cartilage and ligaments can be detected and sometimes repaired through the arthroscope.

4. **Medical History and Examination Evaluation:** A careful analysis of the location, duration and character of the joint symptoms and the appearance of the joints helps the doctor in diagnosing osteoarthritis. Bony

enlargement of the joints from spur formations is characteristic of osteoarthritis.

5. **Other Tests:** Biochemical tests to rule out diabetes, gout etc.

Treatment

1. Weight reduction.
2. Avoiding activities that put pressure on damaged joints.
3. Resting sore joints decreases stress on the joints and relieves pain and swelling.
4. Physical and occupational therapy is very beneficial. Physical therapists can provide support devices, such as splints, canes, walkers and braces.
5. Mechanical support devices. These measures are particularly important when large, weight-bearing joints are involved, such as the hips or knees.
6. Medication may be used topically, taken orally or injected into the joints to decrease joint inflammation and pain.
7. Surgery can be considered when conservative methods fail.
8. Exercise usually does not aggravate osteoarthritis when performed at levels that do not cause joint pain. Exercise is helpful in osteoarthritis in several ways. First, it strengthens the muscular support around the joints. It also prevents the joints from 'freezing up' besides improving and maintaining joint mobility. Finally, it helps with weight reduction and promotes

endurance. Applying local heat before and cold packs after exercise can help relieve pain and inflammation. Swimming is particularly well suited to patients with osteoarthritis because it allows patients to exercise with minimal impact stress to the joints. Other popular exercises include walking, stationary cycling and light weight training.

Chapter 20

Urinary Tract Infection (UTI)

The urinary tract is the body's filtering system for removal of liquid wastes. When bacteria invade and multiply in the urinary tract, UTI occurs. Women are especially susceptible to UTI.

Although most urinary tract infections or UTIs are not serious, they are painful. Approximately 50 per cent of all women have at least one UTI in her lifetime with many women having several infections throughout their lifetime.

The risk for UTIs, both symptomatic and asymptomatic, is highest in women after menopause. Studies indicate that 20 – 25 per cent of women over 65 years of age have UTIs and 10 – 15 per cent will have bacteria in their urine without producing any symptoms. Sexual activity plays a lesser role in UTIs in older women than in younger women. In general, biologic changes due to menopause put older women at particular risk for primary and recurring UTIs:

1. With oestrogen loss, the walls of the urinary tract thin, weakening the mucous membrane and reducing its ability to resist bacteria. The bladder may lose elasticity and fail to empty completely.

2. Oestrogen loss has also been associated with reduction in certain immune factors in the vagina that help block E. coli from adhering to vaginal cells.

3. Levels of lactobacilli (protective bacteria) decline after menopause, perhaps also due to drops in oestrogen levels.

Other age-related urinary conditions, such as urinary incontinence, can increase the risk for recurrent urinary tract infections.

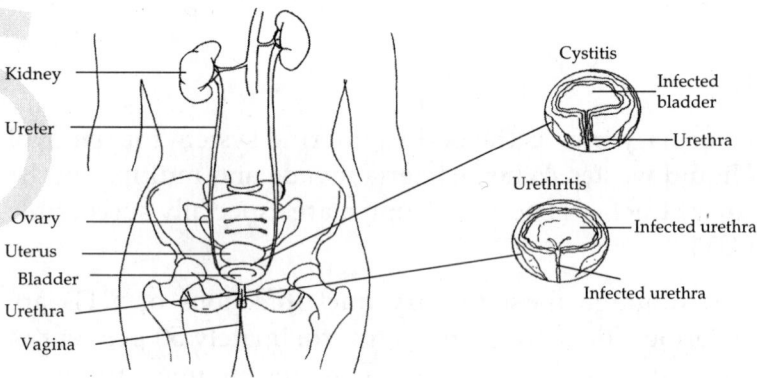

Fig. 20.1: Urinary tract

Medical Conditions That Increase the Risk for UTIs

1. **Diabetes:** Diabetes puts women at significantly higher risk for asymptomatic bacteriuria. The longer a woman has diabetes, the higher the risk. The risk for UTI complications and fungal related infections is also higher in people with diabetes.

2. **Kidney Problems:** Increase the risk of UTI.

3. **AIDS and Immunosuppressed Patients:** Any infection is dangerous in people whose immune systems are damaged and UTIs are no exception.

4. **Sickle Cell Anaemia:** Patients with sickle cell anaemia are particularly susceptible to kidney damage from their disease and UTIs put them at an even greater risk.

5. **Kidney Stones:** In some cases, kidney stones can cause urinary tract obstruction that leads to infection, particularly pyelonephritis. Symptoms of severe urinary tract infection in people with a history of kidney stones may indicate obstruction, which is a serious condition.

6. **Urinary Tract Abnormalities:** Some people have structural abnormalities of the urinary tract that cause urine to stagnate or flow backward into the upper urinary tract. A prolapsed bladder (cystocoele) can result in incomplete urination so that urine collects, creating a breeding ground for bacteria.

Symptoms

1. A strong urge to urinate that cannot be delayed, followed by a sharp pain or burning sensation in the urethra when the urine is released.

2. Most often very little urine is released and the urine that is released may be tinged with blood.

3. The urge to urinate recurs quickly and soreness may occur in the lower abdomen, back or sides.

4. When bacteria enters the ureters and spreads to the kidneys, symptoms such as back pain, chills, fever, nausea and vomiting may occur, as well as the previous symptoms of lower.

Diagnosis

1. **Urine Test:** You will be asked to give a 'clean catch' urine sample by washing the genital area and collecting a 'midstream' sample of urine in a sterile container. This method of collecting urine helps prevent bacteria around the genital area from getting into the sample and confusing the test results. Urine is examined for white and red blood cells and bacteria. Then the bacteria are grown and tested against different antibiotics to see which drug best destroys the bacteria (sensitivity test).

2. **Intravenous Pyelogram:** It is an investigation which gives X-ray images of the bladder, kidneys and ureters. An opaque dye visible on X-ray film is injected into a vein and a series of X-rays is taken. The film shows an outline of the urinary tract, revealing even small changes in the structure of the tract.

3. **Ultrasound:** If you have recurrent infections, your doctor also may recommend an ultrasound exam, which gives pictures from the echo patterns of sound waves bounced back from internal organs.

4. **Cystoscopy:** A cystoscope is an instrument made of a hollow tube with several lenses and light source, which allows the doctor to see inside the bladder from the urethra.

Treatment

1. **Antibiotics:** The choice of and length of treatment depends on the patient's history and the urine tests that identify the offending bacteria. The sensitivity test is especially useful in helping the doctor select

the most effective drug. The drugs most often used to treat routine, uncomplicated UTIs are trimethoprim trimethoprim/sulfamethoxazole, amoxicillin, nitrofurantoin, norflox, ciprofloxacin. Often, a UTI can be cured with one or two days of treatment if the infection is not complicated by an obstruction or other disorder. Still, many doctors ask their patients to take antibiotics for a week or two to ensure that the infection has been cured. Various drugs are available to relieve the pain of UTI.

2. In post-menopausal women who have recurrent urinary tract infection, **local oestrogen hormonal therapy** may be prescribed.

3. A **heating pad** may also help.

4. Most doctors suggest that **drinking plenty of water** helps cleanse the urinary tract of bacteria.

5. During treatment, it is best to avoid coffee, alcohol and spicy foods.

6. **Quit smoking** as it is associated with cancer of urinary bladder. Drink lots of water. Water will flush out your system, preventing the growth of bacteria.

7. **Urinate when you have to**. Ignoring the call of nature can cause your bladder to stretch and weaken. This can prevent the complete emptying of your bladder, leading to infection.

8. **Urinating after sex** washes away any bacteria that were transmitted during intercourse.

9. **Wipe from front to back**. This will prevent bacteria from your rectum being passed to your urethra.

10. Avoid wearing tight clothes, bathing suits or nylon panties for extended periods. They can trap moisture and cause bacteria to collect.

11. Do not use moisturisers, douches or heavily perfumed soaps around your urethra. This can cause irritation and may trap bacteria.

Chapter 21
Thyroid Problems

The thyroid gland is a butterfly shaped gland located in the neck that secretes hormones that are vital to the physiological functions of our body. The thyroid hormone sets the pace at which the bodily functions take place. The functioning of the thyroid gland is largely dependent on iodine. Thyroid hormone levels are controlled by the thyroid stimulating hormone (TSH) produced by the pituitary gland. Problems of thyroid are much more common in women as compared to men and that too in the older age group.

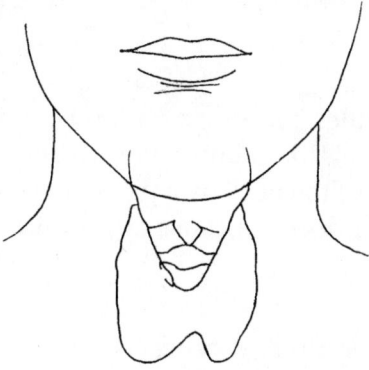

Fig. 21.1: Thyroid gland

Thyroid Problems of Women

Thyroid causes problems for women across all age groups.

Under Active Thyroid (Hypothyroidism)

This condition can occur at any age. It tends to be more common as women get older, particularly after the age of 50 years. Hypothyroidism occurs when the thyroid does not make enough of the thyroid hormone. Symptoms may not be noticeable at first. As the thyroid hormone levels drop, metabolism will begin to suffer as well. A woman who has this problem will begin to feel weak and experience lack of energy. Other symptoms may arise, such as weight gain, menstrual irregularities and constipation.

Overactive Thyroid (Hyperthyroidism)

This is the most common type of thyroid condition in women. It typically occurs in women between the ages of 20 and 40 years. This condition occurs when the thyroid makes too much of the thyroid hormone. Rising hormonal levels increase the metabolism of the body. As a result, the woman will become jittery or irritable, lose weight without even trying to. Sleep problems may also be a part of having an overactive thyroid.

Thyroid Nodules

Sometimes nodules can grow on the side the thyroid and which later on feels like a lump. they can be easily picked up on examination of the neck by a physician. Most of the time, a thyroid nodule does not cause any additional problem.

Thyroid Cancer

The symptoms of thyroid cancer such as pain in the neck and throat or difficulty in swallowing and breathing are sometimes confused with an infection as it usually takes time to reach diagnosis of thyroid cancer. Typical thyroid disease affects women older than 30 years and it can be aggressively seen in older patients. The chances of recovery after treatment of thyroid cancer are more than 95 per cent, if diagnosed and treated in time.

Symptoms

Thyroid symptoms can be noticed in women anytime from puberty to menopause and later. In fact, thyroid disorders can bring about abnormally late or early onset of puberty. Since an overactive or underactive thyroid gland can affect normal ovulation, women suffering from thyroid disease experience problems of temporary infertility. Symptoms of thyroid problem are noticed in about 5 – 8 per cent of women after childbirth. Many a times, thyroid disorder can cause an early onset of menopause. Symptoms of overactive thyroid disorder are often confused with premenopausal symptoms. Symptoms of an underactive thyroid include dry skin, brittle nails, muscle aches and cramps. Depression can also set in. Nearly 20 per cent of chronic cases of depression have been associated with low production of thyroid hormone. Treating thyroid disorders requires just the right amount of medication. Too little thyroid hormone can bring about elevated blood pressure and cholesterol levels. On the other hand, excessive thyroid hormone can increase the risk of bone loss and osteoporosis.

Thyroid Tests

When a thyroid problem is suspected, a thorough medical history and physical examination is conducted. An examination of your neck is done to feel the thyroid gland and any mass on it. Other thyroid tests that might be suggested by a physician are—thyroid ultrasound, blood tests for thyroid and thyroid scan. Thyroid scans are used to test the presence of nodules and also to measure the size of the gland. A thyroid ultrasound test is used to detect if the nodules are solid or fluid-filled cysts. This thyroid test will help in accurately measuring the size of the nodules. It aids in fine needle aspiration biopsy. A fine needle aspiration is conducted on the thyroid gland to take samples of tissues to aid diagnosis of any thyroid disease.

Thyroid Hormones

There are two main thyroid hormones secreted by the thyroid gland—thyroxine and tri-iodotyronine. Thyroid hormones play a key role in certain physiological processes such as growth and metabolism as well as cellular differentiation. The thyroid gland produces a hormone known as calcitonin. The parathyroid glands secrete parathyroid hormone. These thyroid hormones control calcium and phosphorus homoeostasis within the body and affect bone physiology.

Many women suffering from a variety of unresolved symptoms thought to be menopause-related—even when treated with oestrogen—may actually be suffering from undiagnosed thyroid disease. The two conditions often develop in women at the same general age and they often appear at the same time as well. In addition, they share several common symptoms such as, fatigue, mood swings, depression and sleep disturbances. For thyroid, TSH is done and for determining menopause, FSH.

Chapter 22

Mental and Psychological Problems

According to Shirley Chisholm, 'The emotional, sexual and psychological stereotyping of females begins when the doctor says, 'It's a girl'. Many of us will agree with this. Over the years women have been entrusted with more and more diversified roles to play in society. Along with that there have been mounting issues of violence against women, sexual abuse, substance abuse and gender discrimination. As a result depression, anxiety and psychological problems are reported much more commonly in women as compared to men all across the world.

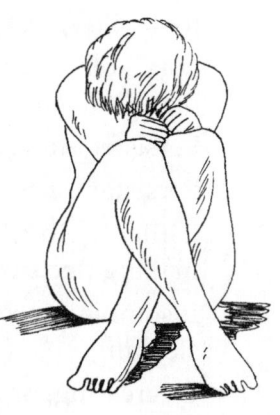

Depression

Everyone occasionally feels blue or sad. These feeling are normal if they occur once in a while as all of us are exposed to different life situations every day. But, when a person is not able to carry out her routine tasks and normal functioning because of this low feeling she is said to be suffering from a depressive disorder. Depression is a common illness which needs to be treated on time as it affects not only the woman but the whole family which is around her and also the productivity at her place of work decreases. Depression on one hand, is more common in women and on the other hand, due to their role and status in society and the stigma attached with mental diseases they are less likely to be taken to a doctor.

Symptoms

1. Feelings of hopelessness and/or pessimism.
2. Feelings of guilt, worthlessness and helplessness.
3. Irritability, restlessness.
4. Loss of interest in activities or hobbies once pleasurable.
5. Persistent fatigue and decreased energy.
6. Persistently sad, anxious or having 'empty' feelings.
7. Difficulty in concentrating, remembering details and making decisions.
8. Insomnia, early morning wakefulness or excessive sleeping.
9. Overeating, or loss of appetite.
10. Thoughts of suicide, suicidal attempts.
11. Persistent aches or pains, headaches, cramps or digestive problems that do not ease even with treatment.
12. Anxiety and phobias generally accompany depression.
13. Alcohol and other substance abuse or dependence may also co-occur with depression.

Probable Causes

It is now believed that depression is caused by a combination of genetic factors and exposure to a stressful life event. There are many causes for clinical depression:

1. It can be inherited that is, the chance of a person having the condition increases considerably if one or more family members have it.
2. Some people have personality traits that make them more susceptible to depression. These people view themselves as losers and have a negative attitude towards themselves.
3. Serious and sensitive personal loss like the death of a near and dear one can cause a depressive episode.
4. Any long duration illness can be followed by depression.
5. Depression can also be a side effect of certain drugs used to treat hypertension.

Women and Depression

What is peculiar about women which makes them more prone to depression? Physical and sexual abuse, poverty, unhappy marriages, hormonal changes over the menstrual cycle, childbirth and menopause and a tendency to focus on depressed feelings rather than taking steps to master them are more common in women. Single parent women, those constantly worried about their physical image and obesity are also under more stress. Besides women face the additional stresses of work and home responsibilities, caring for children and ageing parents.

Diagnosis

Depression, even the most severe cases, is a highly treatable disorder. As with many illnesses, the earlier that treatment can begin, the more effective it is and the greater the likelihood that recurrence can be prevented.

The first step to getting appropriate treatment is to visit a doctor. Certain medications and some medical conditions such as viruses or a thyroid disorder, can cause the same symptoms as depression. A doctor can rule out these possibilities by conducting a physical examination, interview and lab tests. If the doctor can eliminate a medical condition as a cause, he or she should conduct a psychological evaluation or refer the patient to a mental health professional.

Treatment

1. **Anti-depressants**: These are generally given as oral preparation. They have a calming effect on the patient and also help in reducing sleep problems. For all classes of anti-depressants, patients must take regular doses for at least 3-4 weeks before they are likely to experience a full therapeutic effect. The medicine should be stopped only on the advice of the doctor otherwise a relapse may occur. These drugs are not habit forming and are safe to take. Some individuals, such as those with chronic or recurrent depression, may need to stay on the medication indefinitely.

2. **Electro Convulsive Therapy:** This is given in severe cases of depression. It is mostly resorted to when the patient cannot wait for the drugs to become effective, or when she goes into deeper depression and stops reacting completely to situations. Medication should be stopped only under a doctor's supervision. Some medications need to be gradually stopped to give the body time to adjust. Although anti-depressants are not habit forming or addictive, abruptly ending an anti-depressant can cause withdrawal symptoms or lead to a relapse.

3. **Other Medications:** Sometimes stimulants, anti-anxiety medications are prescribed with an anti-depressant, especially if the patient has a co-existing mental or physical disorder. However, neither anti-anxiety medications nor stimulants are effective against depression when taken alone and both should be taken only under a doctor's close supervision.

4. **Psychotherapy**: Talking and counselling the person can help to some extent in case of mild depression but otherwise treatment is most definitely recommended.

Stress and Anxiety

Stress in small doses works like a motivator and energizer but prolonged stress can take a toll on your mental and physical health if you cannot cope with it. High stress levels have been linked to a number of disease conditions like depression, anxiety, cardiovascular disease, musculoskeletal problems, an impaired immune system and cancer. Stress can arise due to various factors such as:

1. **Job Stress:** Women may suffer from mental and physical harassment at work places, apart from the common job stress. Also, subtle discriminations at workplaces, family pressure and societal demands add to these stress factors.

2. **Parental Stress:** 'Nothing describes parenting better than stress!', according to Ron Huxley. Whether the mother is of a newborn, young, old or many children, all are associated with stress. Parenting can be made a pleasurable experience despite stresses associated with it by accepting the fact that stress can't be avoided and by seeking experience from those who have experienced these difficult situations before. Children who are aggressive, substance users, underperforming

in school, hyperactive or chronically ill are difficult to handle. Also, if there is a child in the family who is physically or mentally handicapped or if there are step-children, the situation can be even more stressful. Also it is important that you communicate with your children and encourage them to do the same with you.

3. **Marital Stress:** Not getting married, to being married with an unaffectionate spouse, to divorces, to extramarital affairs—all the relationships are stressful due to the nature of expectations and demands from one another and societal pressures. Not only the relationship but other issues associated with it like living in a joint family and managing the in laws, step-children, financial constraints, etc., all build up a serious situation. It is often that these everyday stresses may manifest as depression, hypertension or anxiety.

4. **Career and Family Life:** Balancing family with professional life is a tricky task. It is important to consider the priorities and evaluate the choices, so that you maintain a balance between all types of activities.

Identify your stress triggers and time management barriers.

Try one or more of these techniques to help identify the factors causing you stress:

   i. Maintain a record for one week, where you note which events and situations cause a negative physical, mental or emotional response. Briefly define the situation, which part of the day did the event occur, who all were involved and how did you perceive it and react to it.

ii. Maintain a record of all the activities you undertake in a day, how much time you spend on each one of them. Whether you need more time with a particular activity or need to do away with an activity all together.

iii. At the work place and at home, set realistic limits, make friends and take regular breaks. When in doubt and trouble seek help. Tasks that can be done by others or have an alternate solution should be tackled accordingly. Try and peruse your favourite hobby and take some time out for physical activity. In case the situation goes out of control, seek professional help. If need be, a sedative will be prescribed to you. If you are fond of pets, it is a very endearing way of distressing. Along with that a healthy diet which provides adequate energy at short intervals should be taken.

Chapter 23

Memory Loss

As we age, we worry about loss of memory. But not all loss of memory is dementia or Alzheimer's disease. Our brain can be kept active with little efforts from our side.

Normal Forgetfulness

The following types of memory lapses are normal among older adults and are generally not considered as warning signs of dementia:

1. Forgetting where you left things you use regularly, such as glasses or keys.
2. Forgetting names of acquaintances or figures in the news.
3. Occasionally forgetting an appointment.
4. Having trouble remembering what you just read.
5. Walking into a room and forgetting why you entered.
6. Forgetting the details of conversations.
7. Becoming easily distracted.
8. Not quite being able to retrieve information easily.

9. Blocking one memory with a similar one, such as calling your one daughter by the other one's name.

10. Mild cognitive impairment.

When you forget things which are not trivial like your marriage anniversary, weekly dance class, etc. then memory loss may be diagnosed as **mild cognitive impairment** (MCI).

The memory lapses are similar to those of someone in the earliest stage of Alzheimer's and some experts see it as a precursor to Alzheimer's or other forms of dementia.

Alzheimer's Disease and other Forms of Dementia

When memory loss becomes so pervasive and severe that it disrupts your work, hobbies, social activities and family relationships, you may be experiencing the warning signs of Alzheimer's disease, another disorder that causes dementia or a condition that mimics dementia. However, the memory problems associated with Alzheimer's disease persist and worsen. While Alzheimer's disease usually affects those over the age of 65 years, a rare and aggressive form of Alzheimer's can happen in some people in their forties and fifties. Alzheimer's disease progresses slowly, taking between 3-18 years to advance from the earliest symptoms to death; the average duration of the disease is 8 years. Death results not from the disease itself but from some secondary illness such as pneumonia or urinary tract infection. Right now, treatment of Alzheimer's disease focuses on slowing its progression and coping with its symptoms.People with Alzheimer's may:

1. Repeat things.

2. Often forget conversations or appointments.

3. Routinely misplace things, often putting them in illogical locations.
4. Eventually forget the names of family members and everyday objects.

Problems with Abstract Thinking

People with Alzheimer's may initially have trouble balancing their checkbook, a problem that progresses to trouble recognising and dealing with numbers.

Difficulty Finding the Right Word

It may be a challenge for those with Alzheimer's to find the right words to express thoughts or even follow conversations. Eventually, reading and writing are also affected.

Disorientation

People with Alzheimer's disease often lose their sense of time and dates and may find themselves lost in familiar surroundings.

Loss of Judgment

Solving everyday problems, such as knowing what to do if food on the stove is burning, becomes increasingly difficult, eventually impossible. Alzheimer's is characterised by greater difficulty in doing things that require planning, decision making and judgment.

Difficulty Performing Familiar Tasks

Once-routine tasks that require sequential steps, such as cooking, become a struggle as the disease progresses.

Eventually, people with advanced Alzheimer's may forget how to do even the most basic things.

Personality Changes

People with Alzheimer's may exhibit:

1. Mood swings.
2. Distrust in others.
3. Increased stubbornness.
4. Social withdrawal.
5. Depression.
6. Anxiety.
7. Aggressiveness.

There are certain conditions which produce memory loss symptoms such as, exposure to lead and mercury. Exposure to pesticides and carbonmonoxide. Certain medications, alcohol and drug abuse can also cause memory loss. Problems of the thyroid, vitamin B12 deficiency and depression can also contribute towards memory loss.

Visit your physician if your memory loss episodes become frequent and noticeable by others. Doctor will take a detailed history and do an examination. If need be, you will be asked to take a mental ability test. If there are problems with this then you will be asked to undergo imaging tests of the brain like CT scan and MRI. If a certain condition is diagnosed then treatment is started.

Compensating for Memory Loss

Even if you are experiencing a troublesome level of memory loss, there are many things you can do to learn new information and retain it.

1. Maintain a day planner and put all the important appointments and tasks to do on it.
2. If you forget how to do a particular activity, write down the steps of the activity.
3. Always put things at the same place be it your watch, or keys, or shoes.
4. Set a reminder to tell you about the appointment.
5. Tell your family members and close friends before leaving home and also of important things to do.
6. If you must drive, always carry a map with you.
7. While going for shopping make a checklist of things to be bought and put a mark against the things purchased.

Preventing Memory Loss

1. **Regular Exercise:** This prevents the onset of diseases like heart disease and diabetes which are associated with memory loss. Exercise also provides more oxygen to the brain.
2. **Diet:** Taking a healthy diet including fruits and vegetables which provide antioxidants help fight memory loss. Vitamin B12 rich diet protects the neurons.
3. **Smoking:** Do not smoke.
4. **Alcohol Consumption:** Do not take alcohol.
5. **Sleep:** Have a sound sleep.
6. **Stress Management:** Try and manage stress and keep it at the lowest level achievable.
7. **Mental Exercise:** Exercise your brain by reading newspaper and magazines, solving a crossword puzzle, learning a new recipe, driving on a new route, pursuing a new hobby, etc.

Chapter 24

Sexual Health

During middle age, sexual intimacy may not be the most vital issue on a person's mind as there are multiple activities to be handled concerning various facets of life.

However, some middle aged women feel at their sexual prime as they are more comfortable with their bodies and independent now whereas some feel it is for the younger population and not an important issue for them. Sexual intimacy is a healthy part of a loving and committed relationship. According to a research in Australia, estimates indicate that about 55 per cent of married women over 60 years and up to 24 per cent of married women over 76 years are sexually active. With increase in life expectancy, physicians are likely to encounter more of sexual problems in the older population.

However, doctors are often uncomfortable talking about sexuality and the topic is ignored in consultations with older patients. While many doctors report that they would be willing to discuss sexuality, if patients initiated the subject, research indicates that older women patients from various settings across the globe are uncomfortable to do so. As the older women in their younger days were brought up in a more conservative society it is not easy for them to open up during old age. Sexual abuses have been common through all the eras but it is only now that some organisations have started speaking openly about them. Women who have unresolved issues related to sexual intimacy should seek professional help to find a solution to their problem.

Perception of the body is also a part of sexuality. Physical perception issues are common for women of all ages and they might not necessarily be accurate. If the way you feel about your body prevents you from doing things you love to do then you can try and change it more to your liking through physical effort, diet, or other reasonable modification. There is nothing wrong in enjoying your sexual life as you age and the guilt should not hold you back from working on it.

Because sexuality tends to be a private matter, it's likely that you've heard less about sexual change than any other element of aging. Fortunately, the news is good—for most healthy adults, pleasure and interests do not diminish with age. Around the age of 50 years, men and women typically begin to notice changes in their sexual drive, sexual response or both. Like so many other physical changes that evolve over time, these aren't signs that you are losing your sexuality. Rather, these changes are simply something to adjust to and discuss openly with your partner and/or your doctor.

Normal Sexual Changes in Women

After menopause, oestrogen, and androgen levels drop, causing physical changes. It can take longer to become sexually excited. Your skin may be more sensitive and easily irritated when caressed. Your sexual drive decreases. Intercourse may be painful because of thinning vaginal walls (regular sex often helps prevent this from becoming severe). If a water-based lubricant is not enough, vaginal estrogen cream can be used which reverses thinning and sensitivity.

It is possible that medication which you are taking for an existing health problem may be hampering enjoyment of a sexually active life. Also a number of health conditions can lead to sexual problems. These concerns need to be discussed with your doctor in detail.

Factors Affecting Sexuality

Physical Causes of Sexual Problems

Physical causes of sexual problems in older women include: Hormonal changes, high blood pressure, high cholesterol levels, heart disease, diminished pelvic blood flow, trauma or surgery, spinal cord injuries diseases of the central or peripheral nervous system.

Psychosocial Factors Affecting Sexuality

The presence or absence of a partner affects the sexual practices of older women. With life expectancy of women exceeding that of men, many older women will eventually live alone and may have limited opportunities for intimate relationships. Also many women suffer from loss of self-esteem as they lose employment, support and mobility. For an older woman who has a partner, the frequency of sexual activity will also be affected by the partner's health status. About 57 per cent of men at the age 60 years have erectile dysfunction, a problem that increases with age. This often has an impact on their partner's expression of sexuality. However, a loving and caring partner will positively encourage the continuation of a sexual relationship.

What can be done?

It is common for women to feel shy discussing their sexual needs and fantasies with their partners. In order to make it easy, one should start talking with the partner. Clearly mention if you have anxiety about some issue. Talk regularly. You can read a book on women's sexual health and recommend your partner to also read it. Issues faced by you for example, lack of time, monotonous sexual routine, what brings pleasure to you and what is uncomfortable, if anything new needs to be experimented should be discussed amply. If there are any rumors, or misbelieves, or myths which are causing a problem then those should be addressed as well. Mismatched sexual desires, effect of alcohol and body changes due to weight gain can also come in the way of sexual pleasure. If a recurrent STI is the issue, discuss that, too. If the talks with your partner are not successful, seek medical help.

Management of Sexual Problems

1. Detailed history of sexual and health problems should be taken.
2. Vulval and pelvic examination should be done.
3. If the lady is on any medication, it needs to be enquired as certain drugs can lead to loss of libido.

Hormonal Treatment

Topical Therapy

Local urogenital symptoms are a common cause of sexual problems in older women. It may be more appropriate in this age group to use topical oestrogen therapy in the form of vaginal pessaries or creams that are not systemically absorbed. A Danish study found that the most common sexual dysfunction in older women was vaginal dryness, which was present in a third of women. Topical oestrogens plus the use of vaginal lubricants relieve dryness associated with vaginal atrophy, which is a common cause of dyspareunia. Topical use of oestrogens may also help to alleviate other urogenital problems, including prolapse of the uterus, cervix, vagina, bladder and rectum and incontinence. Such problems can have physical and emotional effects on older women's sexual well being.

Hormone Replacement Therapy

Long term use of oral, continuous, combined hormonal preparations may be inadvisable in view of the increased risk of breast cancer. However, short-term use (less than 5 years) may alleviate some of the symptoms of oestrogen deficiency. Doses can be titrated according to symptom relief.

The use of tibolone, a synthetic corticosteroid, may also be considered. Studies in post-menopausal women have shown that it can enhance libido and mood and reduce vaginal dryness and consequent dysparunia.

Testosterone Therapy

Testosterone replacement therapy in selected older women may also be considered after appropriate counselling about risks and side effects. Clinical experience has shown that testosterone therapy is helpful for some women who have diminished libido and persistent fatigue with no clear cause. It is usual to use oestrogen with androgen as therapy. Please make sure that the drugs you use have approval for use in your country.

Chapter 25

Pregnancy After 40

Bearing children in the twenties and thirties is what is considered healthy and practiced by most of the women. Also, being able to conceive a child proves a lady's fertility and her status in the family. The thought of having children after the age of 40 years seems discomforting and scary to a lot of us. With passing years we are seeing more and more women bearing children after 40 years of age. The reasons range from demanding careers to having a sound financial status or even late marriage. Conceiving after the age of 40 years is associated with health issues and risks for the mother but for women who conceive after a long struggle, either due to treatment of infertility or have another child due to the death of the previous child—late pregnancies are a source of hope and celebrations, to fulfill their motherhood dreams.

Gradually over the past few years the number of women getting pregnant after the age of 40 has reached a record high after doubling over the past 15 years.

Age and Fertility

Women are born with a total number of eggs for their lifetime. As your age increases, the count of eggs falls and that is the reason why fertility peaks in most women in the twenties and gradually begins to decline in the late twenties. Around the age of 35 years, fertility starts to decline at a much more rapid pace. While we are born with over a million eggs, by puberty just 300,000 are left. From this huge number of eggs, only 300 will ever become mature and be released in the process known as ovulation. Way before menopause begins, our bodies' reproductive capabilities slow down, becoming less effective at producing mature, healthy eggs. As you age and come closer to menopause, your ovaries respond less well to the hormones that are responsible for helping the eggs ovulate. This natural decline of fertility happens in the healthiest of women, though bad health habits, like smoking, have been shown to speed up the decline of fertility. Even the use of in-vitro fertilisation is associated with a poor success rate in older women. Late pregnancy can be associated with many medical illnesses which can have harmful effects, on the foetus and the mother. Medical illnesses affecting the mother and foetus include:

1. Genetic abnormalities and birth defects.
2. Pregnancy loss.
3. Complications of labour and delivery.

Maternal and Child Illnesses

Certain medical conditions occur more frequently in pregnant women over 40, including diabetes, high blood pressure and thyroid disorders. Fortunately, these conditions can be diagnosed and controlled prior to pregnancy and many of the medications used to treat these disorders can be safely used during pregnancy. If you currently take medication and you are planning a pregnancy, talk to your doctor. A change in medication or an adjustment of dosage may be necessary. If not properly treated, maternal illnesses can adversely affect the foetus. Uncontrolled high blood pressure can restrict foetal growth and, in severe cases, can result in stillbirth. Undiagnosed diabetes can carry with it a higher risk of birth defects and poor blood sugar control during pregnancy can result in abnormal foetal growth. Early prenatal care and judicious use of medication can lower these risks significantly.

Genetic Defects

As a woman ages, a higher proportion of her ageing eggs contain chromosomal abnormalities. At the present time, some infertility centers have the technology to weed out these abnormal eggs, but for the majority of women who become pregnant after the age of 40, the risk of a genetic defect increases based on age.

While the general population of child bearing women has a 3 per cent chance of delivering a child with a birth defect, after the age of 40, this risk is between 6 per cent and 8 per cent. The likelihood of having a baby with Down's syndromes approximately 1 in 365 at the age of 35. This number increases to 1 in 100 by the age of 40 and up to 1 in 40 at the age of 45.

Pregnancy Loss

Pregnancy loss also increases with advancing age. Approximately 60 per cent of early (first trimester) miscarriages are due to genetic abnormalities of the foetus. Overall, pregnant women experience miscarriage 15 per cent of the time. After the age of 40, this incidence nearly doubles. There is also a moderate increase in stillbirths after the age of 40 due to a combination of medical complications affecting pregnancy and lethal birth defects.

Complications of Labour and Delivery

Complications of labour and delivery that are seen more frequently in women over the age of 40 include:

1. Premature labour.
2. Premature separation of the placenta resulting in haemorrhage.
3. Placenta praevia (abnormal placement of the placenta over the opening of the cervix).
4. Meconium-stained amniotic fluid (foetal waste in the amniotic fluid which can be harmful if breathed in by the foetal at birth).
5. Postpartum haemorrhage.
6. Malpresentations (breech or other positions other than head down).

As a result, the rate of Cesaream section is considerably higher in this age group.

How to Lower Your Chances of Complications

See Your Doctor

A thorough evaluation prior to pregnancy will allow your doctor to give you an idea of your individual risk. Early prenatal care and good health habits will result in a healthy baby and a happy mother.

Get Healthy

The idea is to be as healthy as you can before you get pregnant. Here are some tips:

1. If you smoke, quit.

2. Avoid alcohol; alcohol can increase the risk of certain birth defects and interfere with proper foetal growth.

3. Avoid caffeine; even moderate caffeine intake might increase your risk of miscarriage (although this remains controversial).

4. Eat a well balanced diet. This means one that is rich in fruits, vegetables, whole grains and low fat dairy and other protein sources. Start a prenatal vitamin prior to pregnancy and stick with it. The folic acidin prenatal vitamins is known to reduce certain birth defects and the iron supplement will combat anaemia.

5. Perform moderate amount of exercise. Exercise is good for toning muscles and limbering joints, thereby decreasing the normal aches and pains associated with pregnancy. If you are not exercising already, check with your doctor before starting an exercise program.

Get Tested

1. Blood tests are available to screen for some genetic disorders; a 'triple screen' or 'quad screen' blood test may be obtained to evaluate the risk of neural tube defects and Down's syndrome.

2. Genetic amniocentesis (or chorionic villus sampling) is offered to women after the age of 35. Amniocentesis is usually done in the third or fourth month of pregnancy and involves removal of amniotic fluid from the womb for genetic testing. There is a minimal (0.25 per cent)

risk of miscarriage associated with this test. This risk is outweighed however by the slightly larger risk of having an undetected abnormality.

3. Chorionic villus sampling can be done earlier in pregnancy and involves the removal of a minute amount of placental tissue, which can then be tested for genetic abnormalities. The risk of miscarriage may be as high as 0.75 – 1.0 per cent with this test.

Despite the real, perceived or potential risks, all studies agree that the actual outcome for the baby is every bit as good as that for younger mothers, as shown by the Apgar scores which assess a baby's well being immediately after birth and the on-going checks through childhood. On the psychological front, older mothers may again have an advantage. One study shows that they have less fear of helplessness and loss of control than younger women. Also the years can give greater stamina and courage.

Many women who want to become pregnant again after a tubal ligation are over 35 years of age and want to know what their chances are of having another baby. Although doctors often give pessimistic opinions about this, the Tubal Reversal Study at Chapel Hill Tubal Reversal Center gives encouraging news for these women. Among women aged 35 – 39 years, the pregnancy rate was 58 per cent and for women 40 years and older, the pregnancy rate was 40 per cent. Although these rates are lower than for younger women, they show that as long as a woman is still ovulating, pregnancy is still possible regardless of age.

With all the advances in medical care and technology, it is safer today than ever before for most women in later age to become pregnant.

Chapter 26

Contraception After 40

A woman's fertility declines slowly with age after the age of 30. It drops by 50 per cent, by the age of 40 years. Contraception is still an important issue at this age as pregnancy at this age could be unwanted and also associated with more health problems for the mother and child. This is the time to re-evaluate one's contraceptive choice depending upon one's requirement of effectiveness of the contraceptive, need for protection from sexually transmitted diseases, side effects and reduction in heavy bleeding.

Methods of Contraception

Sterilisation

Sterilisation is a permanent method of contraception and hence reassures a woman. Male sterilisation or **vasectomy** involves cutting and tying, or blocking the tubes (the vas deferens) that carry sperms from the testicles to the penis. The procedure is performed through either a small incision in the scrotum or a 'no-scalpel' method and usually it only requires a local anaesthetic. It can be done as a day surgery or in a medical specialist's office. Vasectomy has no effect on sexual drive, erection, or ejaculation. Side effects include bruising and discomfort for a few days after the procedure. A small percentage of men develop chronic pain which reduces over time. Vasectomy is a very popular option in Australia with the rate 5 times higher than that of tubal ligation.

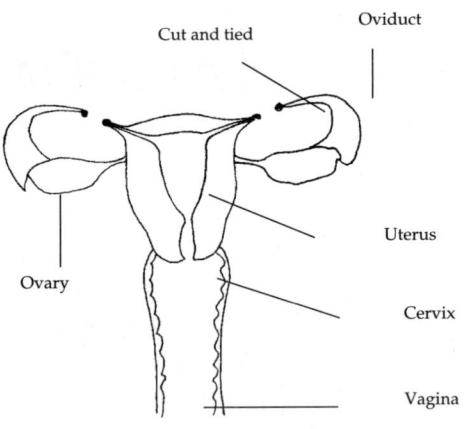

Fig 26.1.: Tubal ligation

Female sterilisation or **tubal ligation** (Fig. 26.1) involves blocking fallopian tubes by cutting or burning, or by the use of clips, clamps or rings. Tubal ligation is most commonly performed as a laparoscopic procedure under general anaesthesia. Laparoscopy involves one to three small incisions near the navel. The abdomen is filled with gas and a laparoscope, an instrument that allows the interior of the abdomen to be viewed, is inserted through one of the incisions. Tubal ligation has no effect on sexual drive or on the menstrual cycle. It usually takes about a week after surgery for the abdominal discomfort caused by the gas to subside. Tubal ligation carries the risks associated with surgery and anaesthesia. Vasectomy is not effective immediately, so another form of contraception must be used in the interim for 3 months. If a woman does become pregnant after female sterilisation there is a higher risk the pregnancy will be ectopic (in the fallopian tubes).

A new female sterilisation procedure, **Essure**, is now available. It involves the insertion of a small flexible device called a 'micro-insert' into each of the fallopian tubes causing scar tissue to form, blocking the tubes. The Essure procedure requires no incisions (instead, access is via the vagina/cervix) and can usually be performed under local anaesthesia.

There are now reversible methods of contraception available which have failure rates as low as sterilisation (that is, implanon, intrauterine system). These may provide a suitable alternative to permanent methods for some women.

Combined Oral Contraceptive Pill

The combined oral contraceptive pill consists of a combination of the hormones oestrogen and progestogen. In the past, it was often recommended that women only take the pill until the age of 35 years. The lower dosages used today, however, allow women who have no risk factors for heart disease and are non-smokers to continue on this form of contraception until menopause.

The pill can provide women with a number of benefits in addition to effective contraception. Irregular cycles, commonly experienced in the perimenopause may be controlled with the pill, as can heavy or painful periods. The use of the pill is also associated with a reduced incidence of gynaecological disorders such as pelvic infection, ovarian cysts and cancer of the ovaries and uterus. Perimenopausal symptoms such as, hot flushes and vaginal dryness may also be reduced with the pill. Women should be given the lowest effective dose. Side effects like breast enlargement, tenderness, nausea, slightly increased risk of breast cancer need to be considered.

Progestogen Only Pill (POP) or Mini Pill

POP is a good choice for older women as its effectiveness is comparable to that of the pill in young women. The progestogen only pill consists of low doses of the synthetic hormone progesterone. Women who are unable to take the pill (breast feeding, smokers, family history of blood clots), or who experience unpleasant side effects from its oestrogen component, may be able to take POP. POP must be taken at the same time every day, with a pill being considered 'missed' if it is more than three hours late. Side effects include irregular menstrual bleeding, sometimes with nuisance spotting. Less commonly, amenorrhoea, headaches and breast tenderness may occur.

Condoms

Condoms offer effective contraception if used properly and consistently at the same time. They can also protect against sexually transmitted diseases. Lubricated condoms or the use of an additional lubricant can be helpful for women who are experiencing vaginal dryness. Female condoms are non-latex (polyurethane) so an oil-based lubricant can be used. For people with latex allergies, polyurethane male condoms are available. Only water-based lubricants should be used with male condoms as petroleum or oil-based lubricants (like, vaseline and baby oil) can damage the latex, causing it to break.

Condoms may not be acceptable to women who have not regularly used them in the past. Some couples feel that there is a reduction in sensation when using condoms and women may also experience allergies to the latex in the male condom or to the lubricants used. Maintaining an erection is a problem experienced by some older men who use condoms.

Intrauterine Contraceptive Device (IUCD)

The intrauterine contraceptive device (IUCD) is a small, flexible device, made from plastic and copper, which is inserted into the uterus via the cervix. An IUCD fitted when a woman is over 40 years can actually remain in place until menopause. The risk of expulsion, where the IUCD is completely or partially pushed out of the uterus, is lower in older women. IUCDs can be left inside the uterus for about 5 years.

The intrauterine system (IUS), called **Mirena,** differs from conventional IUCDs in that it has a stem which releases a steady low dose of progesterone. Besides providing contraception, Mirena has the added benefit of greatly reducing a woman's menstrual flow by making the lining of the uterus (endometrium) very thin. This feature makes Mirena ideal for women who experience menstrual problems like heavy bleeding. It lasts for 5 years. Women who have more then one sexual partner and are at an increased risk of sexually transmitted diseases should not use theses contraceptive devices.

Side effects of IUCD may include heavier, longer or more painful periods. Side effects of Mirena may include irregular bleeding or amenorrhoea. Other typical progesterone-related side effects (breast tenderness, headaches, acne and mood changes) are less common with Mirena as the amount of progesterone is small.

Diaphragm

The diaphragm is a soft, dome-shaped rubber cap which fits across the vagina, covering the cervix to block the sperms. It is fitted prior to intercourse and needs to stay in place for longer than 6 hours after the last time vaginal sex occurred. Diaphragms are often used in conjunction with a spermicide.

A lady should learn how to fit the diaphragm under the supervision of a doctor initially as they may find it difficult to fit it. Some women may experience an allergic reaction to the rubber or spermicide. Diaphragms are associated with a slightly increased risk of urinary tract infections and are unsuitable for women with pelvic floor weakness and/or genital prolapse.

Progestogen Injections and Implants

Medroxyprogesterone acetate or DMPA is a progestogen based. contraceptive given to women as an injection every twelve weeks.

The progestogen implant is a small rod approximately 4 cms long and 2 mm wide. It is inserted under the skin in the upper arm by a medical practitioner with special training in the procedure. It releases a low steady dose of progestogen and lasts for 3 years. Return of normal fertility is delayed on an average for 10 weeks after the last injection. DMPA is associated with a small loss of bone density which is usually reversible after the injections are stopped. 50 per cent of women using DMPA have amenorrhoea after using it for one year. Most women using Implanon have little or no bleeding but 30 per cent may have frequent or prolonged bleeding. Other side effects of both DMPA and implants include weight gain, loss of libido and mood changes.

Withdrawal Method

This involves the withdrawal of the penis completely from the vagina before ejaculation. Even if the penis is withdrawn in time, there is often pre-ejaculate fluid and this can contain some sperms. The effectiveness of this method in the general population (not specifically women over 40 years), ranges from 81-96 per cent, which is greater than not using any contraceptive method. While some couples will find the failure rate unacceptable, others may be comfortable with this level of risk.

Natural Family Planning Methods

These methods involve determining fertile and non-fertile days and abstaining from vaginal sex at 'unsafe' times. While natural methods can be effective for motivated, younger women with regular cycles, they are problematic in women over 40. Irregular cycles and hormonal fluctuations in women this age make calculating the 'safe' days more difficult.

Emergency Contraception

If contraception fails or is overlooked, emergency contraception can be used as a back-up method. There are two forms of emergency contraception available—the IUCD and the emergency contraceptive pill. When inserted within 5 days of unprotected sex, an IUCD will prevent pregnancy and provide ongoing contraception for suitable women. The emergency contraceptive pill can be taken within 72 hours of unprotected sex. It consists of 2 higher dose progestogen tablets, taken 12 hours apart. These pills are available over the counter.

When to Stop Contraception

Women approaching menopause are often unsure of when it is safe to stop the use of contraception. Generally, it is recommended that if a woman is 50 years or younger she should continue using contraception for 2 years following the last menstruation. If she is older than 50, contraception should be used for one year following the last menstruation.

While these guidelines are relevant to women using non-hormonal contraception (condom, diaphragm, IUD), other women will find that the hormones in their contraception will mask the end of their menstruation. For example, the bleeding that a pill user has during the non-active pill week is not a true menstrual period and will continue even after menopause. Similarly, POP and implant users may experience amenorrhoea which will disguise the true end of their menstruation.

For women using hormonal contraceptives, options include:

1. **POP and Implant Users:** Can continue using the contraception until they reach an age where the natural loss of fertility is very likely to have occurred that is, about 55 years of age.

2. **Pill Users:** Can switch to a form of non-hormonal contraception to see if menstruation returns. If menstruation does not return they can then follow the general guidelines for stopping contraception (2 years after last menstruation for those 50 years and under one year after last menstruation for over 50 years old). If menstruation does return, they could either switch back to their hormonal contraceptive and repeat the process at a later date, or continue using the non-hormonal contraception. After the age of 50 years, the use of oral contraceptive pills is not required.

Chapter 27

Physical Fitness

Advances in science, modernisation and industrialisation have made our lives simpler. Daily routines and chores which once took a lot of time and calories away from us have both become a boon and a curse. Our daily expenditure of calories has decreased coupled with an increased availability of a variety of refined food items which please the palate more. If one does not follow a regular exercise routine and obtain a balance in life then the famous saying that 'those who think they have not time for bodily exercise will sooner or later have to find time for illness' will become applicable. As per a research, more than 60 per cent of women do not get the recommended amount of physical activity and 1 in 4 women aren't physically active at all. That number jumps in women over 55 years—nearly 40 per cent of whom say they get no leisure time physical activity.

Benefits of Physical Activity

Physical activity helps to reduce weight and prevent weight gain. Women tend to lose muscle mass and gain abdominal fat during and after menopause. Even a slight increase in physical activity can help prevent weight gain. Physical activity during and after menopause that results in weight loss offers protection from breast cancer and strengthens the bones which lowers the risk of fractures and osteoporosis. The risk of various chronic conditions—including cardiovascular disease and type 2 diabetes—increases. Regular physical activity can decrease these risks. It is a good way to fight depression as well.

Understand your Body to Plan an Exercise Routine

1. **Give Breaks Between Workouts:** As the body ages, it requires more of breaks in between workouts. Do intense workouts and take longer breaks so that your muscles recover and grow.

2. **Loss of Muscle Mass:** Progressive resistance training should be incorporated in your schedule so that the muscle mass drop which occurs with age is compensated for.

3. **Loss of Bone Density:** Begins in the mid thirties. Cardiovascular workout along with resistance training done on a daily basis will prevent bone loss and hence osteoporosis. Fun activities like dancing, walking and playing outdoor games can be incorporated 3-5 times per week. Variety is the spice of life. Avoid routine, monotonous activity; instead try out what you consider is fun for you.

4. **Metabolic Rate Decreases:** Fewer calories are needed to support the same level of activity. Consume complex carbohydrates instead of simple ones. Oats, brown rice and sweet potatoes are fine examples of complex carbohydrates. The problem with simple carbohydrates is after you consume them, there is a sudden rise in the level of insulin, as a result of which you feel hypoglycaemic and feel like eating more.

Enjoy a diet filled with green vegetables—they provide a negative calorie balance that is where more calories are expended to digest the food item than the item itself. Protein levels should be relatively high to support the muscle building process. Lean protein sources include grilled chicken, fish and beef.

5. **Range of Motion Diminishes:** With age, joints stiffen and elasticity is lost in tendons and ligaments resulting in a less flexible body. Yoga, through gentle stretches and daily practice produces a more flexible body.

6. **Hormonal Fluctuations:** Hormonal fluctuations occur during and around menopause. A longer or faster cardiovascular workout to the mix will help prevent the onset of middle age obesity. Feel good hormone—endorphins will also help you fight mood swings.

7. **Watch Out Against Injuries:** As the flexibility decreases with age, chances of injuries increase. Hence, take adequate rest and let the minor injuries heal before you continue with your routine.

Physical Activity Goals

For most healthy women, the Department of Health and Human Services recommends:

1. At least 2 hours and 30 minutes of moderate intensity aerobic activity or 1 hour and 15 minutes of vigorous intensity aerobic activity a week, preferably spread throughout the week.

2. Strength training exercises at least twice a week.

Although frequent, high intensity physical activity during and after menopause may yield the maximum health benefits, it's more important to choose a fitness programme that you can maintain for the long term. Set realistic and achievable goals and depending on your strength and endurance levels, update them timely.

Forms of Physical Activity You Can Undertake

Always consult a physician for a baseline profile of your physical health status before you start exercising.

1. **Aerobic Activity:** Try walking, jogging, biking, swimming or water aerobics. Any physical activity that uses large muscle groups and increases your heart rate counts. If you are a beginner, start with ten minutes of light activity and gradually increase the intensity of your activity.

2. **Strength Training:** Regular strength training can help you reduce your body fat, strengthen your muscles and more efficiently burn calories. Try weight machines, hand-held weights or resistance tubing. Choose a weight or resistance level heavy enough to tire your muscles after about 12 repetitions. Gradually increase the resistance level as you get stronger.

3. **Stretching:** Stretching increases flexibility, improves range of motion and promotes better circulation. Stretching can even relieve stress. Set aside time to stretch after each workout, when your muscles are warm and receptive to stretching. Activities such as yoga promote flexibility too.

4. **Stability and Balance:** Balance exercises improve stability and can help prevent falls. Try simple exercises, such as standing on one leg. Activities such as Tai chi can be helpful too.

A combination of the above mentioned activities is best for you.

General Physical Activites Defined by Level of Activity in Accordance with CDC Guidelines

Moderate Activity by CDC (CENTER FOR DISEASE CONTROL, ATLANTA)

One MET (Ratio of exercise metabolic rate) is defined as the energy expenditure for sitting quietly, which, for the average adult, approximates 3.5 ml of oxygen uptake per kilogram of body weight per minute (1.2 kcal/min for a 70-kg individual). For example, a 2-MET activity requires two times the metabolic energy expenditure of sitting quietly.

Walking at a moderate or brisk pace of 3 to 4.5 mph on a level surface inside or outside, such as:

- Walking to class, work, or the store.
- Walking for pleasure.
- Walking the dog.
- Walking as a break from work.
- Waking downstairs or down a hill.
- Race walking—less than 5 mph.
- Using crutches.
- Hiking.
- Roller skating or in-line skating at a leisurely pace.
- Bicycling 5 to 9 mph, level terrain or with few hills.
- Stationary bicycling—using moderate effort.
- Aerobic dancing—high impact.
- Water aerobics.

- Calisthenics–high impact.
- Yoga.
- Gymnastics.
- General home exercises, light or moderate effort, getting up and down from the floor.
- Jumping on a trampoline.
- Using a stair climber machine at a light-to-moderate pace.
- Using a rowing machine–with moderate effort.
- Weight training and bodybuilding using free weights, Nautilus or Universal-type weights.
- Boxing–punching bag.
- Ballroom dancing.
- Volleyball–competitive.
- Playing frisbee.
- Juggling.
- Curling.
- Cricket–batting and bowling.
- Badminton.
- Archery (non-hunting).
- Fencing.
- Downhill sking–with light effort.
- Ice skating at a leisurely pace (9 mph or less).
- Snowmobiling.

- Ice sailing.
- Swimming–recreational.
- Treading water–slowly, moderate effort.
- Diving–springboard or platform.
- Aquatic aerobics.
- Waterskiing.
- Snorkeling.
- Surfing, board or body.
- Canoeing or rowing a boat at less than 4 mph.
- Rafting–white water.
- Sailing–recreational or competition.
- Paddle boating.
- Kayaking–on a lake, calm water.
- Washing or waxing a powerboat or the hull of a sailboat.
- Fishing while walking along a riverbank or while wading in a stream–wearing waders.
- Hunting deer, large or small game.
- Bathtub while on hands and knees, hanging laundry on a clothesline, sweeping an outdoor area, cleaning out the garage, washing windows, moving light furniture, packing or unpacking boxes, walking and putting household items away, carrying out heavy bags of trash or recyclables (for example, glass, newspapers and plastics), or carrying water or firewood.

- General household tasks requiring considerable effort.
- Putting groceries away – walking and carrying especially large or heavy items less than 50 lbs.
- Actively plying with children–walking, running, or climbing while playing with children walking while carrying a child weighing less than 50 lbs.
- Child care–handling uncooperative young children (for example chasing, dressing, lifting into car seat), or handling several young children at one time.
- Bathing and dressing an adult.
- Animal care–shoveling grain, feeding farm animals, or grooming animals.
- Waiting tables or institutional dishwashing.
- Driving or maneuvering heavy vehicles (for example, semi-truck, school bus, tractor, or harvester)–not fully automated and requiring extensive use of arms and legs.
- Operating heavy power tools (for example, electrical work, plumbing, carpentry, dry wall and painting).
- Farming–feeding and grooming animals, milking cows, shoveling grain, picking fruit form trees, or picking vegetables.
- Packing boxes for shipping or moving.
- Assembly-line work–task requiring movement of the entire body, arms or legs with moderate effort.
- Mail carriers–walking while carrying a mailbag.
- Patient care–bathing, dressing and moving patients, or physical therapy.

Barriers to Physical Exercise

Women face a number of barriers when it comes to starting a daily exercise routine. Not having enough time to devote to fitness seems to be a common barrier. Some have this wrong notion that if they are not obese they need not exercise. Certain others feel they won't be able to cope up with physical activity. Make exercise a part of your daily routine as, 'Motivation is what gets you started. Habit is what keeps you going'.

Chapter 28

Diet

When you are eating healthy you have enough energy to work, feel good and at the same time keep healthy without unnecessarily starving yourself. As suggested by WHO, after the age of 40 years energy requirements in the food should be decreased by 5 per cent per each decade till 60 and then by 10 per cent for each decade thereafter as our metabolism slows down and also the physical activity decreases. If you know the basic vocabulary used in terms of nutrition, you can formulate your own healthy eating plans. Let us get familiar with some of the commonly used terms in relation to nutrition.

Carbohydrates (Carbs)

1. **Bad Carbs:** These are the food items that no longer have fibre and nutrients as they have been removed. Food items are usually processed in order to make cooking fast and easy. Examples are white flour, refined sugar and white rice. They digest quickly causing spikes in blood sugar, which over time can lead to weight gain, hypoglycaemia, or even diabetes.

2. **Good Carbs:** This keeps your blood sugar and insulin levels from rising and falling too quickly, helping you get full quicker and feel fuller longer as they are digested more slowly. Good sources of carbs include whole grains, beans, fruits and vegetables, which also offer lots of additional health benefits, including heart disease and cancer prevention.

Proteins

1. A **complete protein** source is one that provides all of the essential amino acids. Examples are animal based foods such as meat, poultry, fish, milk, eggs and cheese.
2. An **incomplete protein** source is one that is low in one or more of the essential amino acids.
3. **Complementary proteins** are two or more incomplete protein sources that together provide adequate amounts of all the essential amino acids. For example, rice and dry beans. Similarly, dry beans and rice both each are incomplete proteins, but together, these two foods can provide adequate amounts of all the essential amino acids your body needs.

Fats

1. **Saturated fats,** primarily found in animal sources including red meat and whole milk dairy products, raise the low density lipoprotein (LDL or 'bad') cholesterol that increases your risk of coronary heart disease (CHD). Sources of saturated fats of vegetable origin include vegetable oils such as coconut oil, palm oil and foods made with these oils.
2. **Trans fats** are created by heating liquid vegetable oils in the presence of hydrogen gas, a process called **hydrogenation**. Primary sources of trans fat are

vegetable shortenings, some margarine, crackers, candies, cookies, snack foods, fried foods, baked goods and other processed foods made with partially hydrogenated vegetable oils.

3. **Monounsaturated fats** are those whose primary sources are plant oils like canola oil, peanut oil and olive oil. Other good sources are avocados, nuts such as almonds, hazelnuts and seeds such as pumpkin and sesame seeds. Mediterranean diets have high content of these fats.

4. **Polyunsaturated fats** include the omega-3 and omega-6 groups of fatty acids which your body can't make. Omega-3 fatty acids are found in very few foods—primarily cold water fatty fish and fish oils. Foods rich in omega-3 fats can reduce cardiovascular disease, improve your mood and help prevent dementia. As you grow old your metabolism slows down. The following food items can help boost it up for you:

Whole Grain Cereals, Oatmeal

The complex carbohydrates and high fibres in whole grain cereals help boost your metabolism naturally by slowing down the release of insulin. The lower production of insulin helps to keep your metabolism going.

When there is an increase of insulin production in the system, your body receives a signal to start storing food as fat. The metabolism must be slowed down in order for your body to store this fat and therefore you are burning fewer calories during this time. So by eating these metabolism boosting foods, you will slow down the production of insulin and increase your metabolism. Everyone knows that high fibre foods, which include whole grains, oats and brown rice, are essential for a healthy digestive system.

Research has also shown that whole grains offer protection against diabetes, heart disease, stroke, colon cancer, high blood pressure and gum disease. Whole grains also have a lot of vitamins, minerals and (again) fibre compared to their refined versions. Whole grains are the best foods to keep you energised, slim and avoid both short and long term health problems.

Low Fat Yoghurt, Skimmed Milk

Research has shown that those people who included 3 to 4 servings of dairy products in their weight loss plan lost significantly more weight than those who did not include dairy or either had a low dairy intake. Yoghurt is also known to be good for your digestive system, keeping you regular and healthy. Yoghurt is a rich source of calcium, which is vital for both strength and growth. When women enter their middle ages their bones stop strengthening and start deteriorating. Yoghurt and other calcium rich foods such as dairy products, spinach or calcium fortified soy milk. Are very beneficial at this stage. Yoghurt is your best bet as it contains friendly probiotics which keep your gut healthy. Aim to consume at least 700 mg of calcium a day.

Green Tea, Coffee

Green tea is the latest and greatest item that is being advertised as one of the best weight loss foods. Green tea has a component called Epigallo catechin gallate, or EGCG. It is this compound that is believed to be the main ingredient that helps boost your metabolism and aid in weight loss.

Additionally, both green tea and coffee have caffeine. Caffeine speeds up your heart and the faster your heart beats the faster your metabolism. Caffeine has also been shown to increase concentration.

Grapefruit, Oranges

Vitamin C is the secret ingredient to these metabolism booster foods and is said to have some fat burning qualities. Oranges and grapes are its rich sources.

Jalapeno, Habanera, Cayenne

By including these hot peppers in your foods you are boosting your metabolism. This is because they have a thermagenic property which heats up your body. To cool down your body requires calories, meaning an increase in your metabolism.

Lean Turkey, Pork, Chicken and Beef

Protein requires more effort to digest than carbs or fat. This means your body is working harder to digest the protein in these metabolism booster foods and is burning more calories.

Salmon, Tuna Fish

Eating foods containing omega-3 essential fatty acids is essential for brain health. Fish such as salmon, sardines, herring, trout and tuna all contain omega-3. The fatty acids in fish help to control chronic inflammation as they have potent anti-inflammatory effects. Also, many studies have suggested that eating omega-3 fats improve mood as well as attitude and can help beat depression. This in turn will make you feel healthier and full of energy. If you can take two servings you will feel the difference. Omega-3 fatty acids can lower the level of a hormone in your body called leptin. Higher levels of leptin means more foods stored as fat, or a lower metabolism. But lower levels of leptin means a higher metabolism and fish is a great way to lower your leptin. Another healthy note on omega-3 it is also shown to reduce the risk of certain cancers.

Vegetables

Vegetables are a great source for low calorie foods that help satisfy you and make you feel full. Veggies contain fibre, vitamins and nutrients that help keep us healthy. Certain vegetables also are great metabolism booster foods such as broccoli and spinach.

Spinach contains magnesium which has been known to boost the body's fat burning process. Other foods high in magnesium include peanut butter, tofu, whole wheat bread and dark chocolate.

Spinach is also high in potassium which aids weight loss by keeping the body's cells hydrated. If your cells are not sufficiently hydrated, your metabolism will slow down. Other potassium rich foods include bananas, honeydew and baked potatoes. Vegetables get their bright colours thanks to high antioxidant levels. Antioxidants eat up free radicals, which are highly reactive oxygen molecules that damage cells and contribute to skin problems, such as dryness and wrinkles. Therefore vegetables top up the skin's supply of antioxidants, getting rid of free radical whenever they appear. Vegetables also supply a lot of vitamins, minerals and fibre which are all essential for a healthy body. Aim for at least 5 servings of vegetables a day.

Apples, Pears

These low calorie, high fibre fruits are why these are included on the metabolism booster foods list. These fruits will give you a satisfying sweet taste and help to keep you full longer due to the lower calorie and higher fibre content than other fruits.

According to one study from the State University of Rio de Janeiro, women who included apples and pears in their low calorie diet lost more weight than the women who did not add fruit to their weight loss plan.

Water

We should not forget that water is an essential component of our diet. Studies are now showing that water can also help to boost your metabolism. Consume approximately 8 to 10 oz a day.

Nuts

When you get a hunger pang in between meals try taking a handful of nuts, about 20. Nuts have monounsaturated fats which studies have shown help stimulate fat burning as well.

Say No to Alcohol

Alcohol lowers your activity metabolism and can stimulate your appetite. Additionally too much alcohol tends to cloud your mind and in this state you can make the wrong choices like eating too much of the wrong foods.

Avoid

Fruit juices can contain up to 10 teaspoons of sugar per cup; avoid or dilute with water. Canned fruit often contains sugary syrup and dried fruit, while being an excellent source of fibre, can be high in calories. Avoid fried veggies or ones smothered in dressings or sauces—you may still get the vitamins, but you'll be getting a lot of unhealthy fat and extra calories as well.

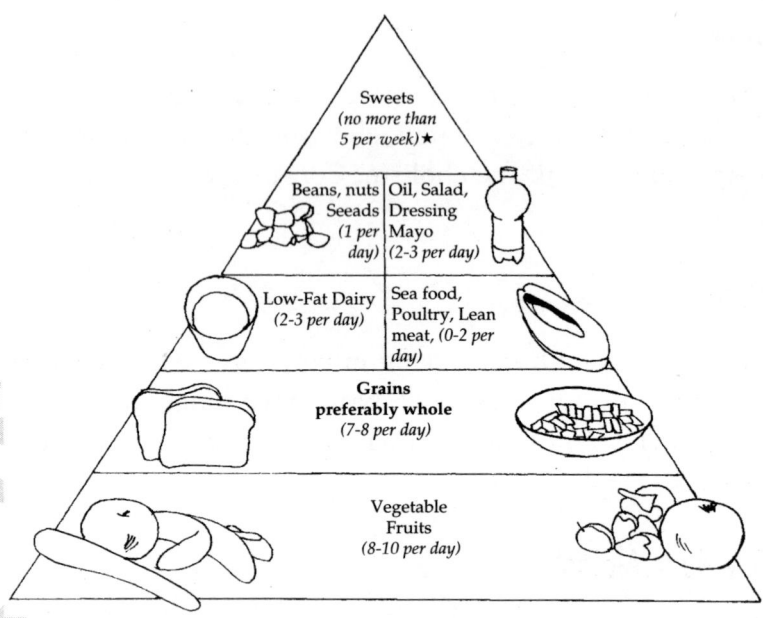

Fig. 28.1: Dash diet – the key to boost women's heart health

Dietary Tips for Diabetes Control

For diabetics, it is essential that they do not starve themselves and at the same time take a well balanced and nutritious diet. This is possible with a meal plan. If you fix the serving size you will be eating an approximately equal amount for all the meals.

For initials tips on diet control after having been diagnosed with diabetes consult a dietician.

A dietitian can provide you valuable information on how to change your eating habits and help you meet goals such as:

1. Controlling overeating.

2. Making better food choices.

3. Losing weight.

If you are taking insulin, he or she can teach you how to count the amount of carbohydrates in each meal or snack and adjust your insulin dose accordingly.

Carbohydrates should account for 45 to 65 per cent of daily calories, proteins for 15 per cent to 20 per cent of the daily calories and fats 20 to 35 per cent. **Eat healthy carbohydrates.** During digestion, sugars (simple carbohydrates) and starches (complex carbohydrates) break down into blood sugar. Focus on the healthiest carbohydrates:

1. Fruits.
2. Vegetables.
3. Whole grains.
4. Legumes (beans, peas and lentils).
5. Low fat dairy products.

Choose Fibre Rich Foods

Dietary fibre includes all parts of plant foods that your body can not digest or absorb. Fibre can decrease the risk of heart disease and help control blood sugar levels. Aim for 25 to 30 grams of fibre each day. Foods high in fibre include:

1. Vegetables.
2. Fruits.
3. Legumes (beans, peas and lentils).
4. Whole wheat flour
5. Wheat bran.
6. Nuts.

Limit Saturated and Trans Fats

Diabetes increases your risk of heart disease and stroke by accelerating the development of clogged and hardened arteries. That is why heart-healthy eating becomes a part of your diabetic diet. Get no more than 7 per cent of your daily calories from saturated fat and try to avoid trans fat completely. The best way to reduce the amount of saturated and trans fats you eat is to:

1. **Limit Solid Fats:** Reduce the amount of butter, margarine and shortening in your diet.
2. **Use Low Fat Substitutions:** For example, top your baked potato with salsa or low-fat yogurt rather than butter. Try sugar free fruit spread on toast instead of margarine.

Choose Monounsaturated and Polyunsaturated Fats

Aim for monounsaturated fats—such as olive oil or canola oil. Polyunsaturated fats found in nuts and seeds, are a healthier choice as well. But moderation is essential. Curb dietary cholesterol. When there's too much cholesterol in your blood, you may develop fatty deposits in your blood vessels. Eventually, these deposits make it difficult for enough blood to flow through your arteries. To help keep your cholesterol under control, consume no more than 200 mg of cholesterol a day.

To reduce cholesterol, eat:

1. Lean cuts of meat instead of organ meats.
2. Egg substitutes over egg yolks.
3. Skimmed milk over whole milk products.

Eat heart-healthy fish atleast twice a week.

Fish can be a good alternative to high fat meats. Cod, tuna and halibut, for example, have less total fat, saturated fat and cholesterol than meat and poultry. Fish such as salmon, mackerel and herring are rich in omega-3 fatty acids, which promote heart health by lowering blood fats called triglycerides.

Using Exchange Lists

A dietitian may recommend using the exchange system, which groups foods into categories such as starches, fruits, meats and meat substitutes and fats.

One serving in a group is called an 'exchange'. An exchange has about the same amount of carbohydrates, protein, fat and calories—and the same effect on your blood sugar—as a serving of every other food in the same group. So, for example, you could exchange or trade either of the following for one carbohydrate serving:

1. 1 small apple
2. 1/3 cup of cooked pasta

Exchange List—Fats

Fats come in various types. Unsaturated fats—including monounsaturated fats and polyunsaturated fats—are healthy if eaten in small amounts. But saturated fats and trans fats can increase your risk of heart disease.

Some people who have diabetes use the glycaemic index to select foods, especially carbohydrates. Foods with a high glycaemic index are associated with a greater increase in blood sugar than are foods with a low glycaemic index. However, low index foods are not necessarily healthier. Foods that are high in fat tend to have lower glycaemic index values than do some healthier options.

Remember these guidelines for including fruits in your diabetes diet:

1. Eat a whole fruit when you can. It has more fibre and is more filling than fruit juice.
2. Select canned fruit and fruit juices without added sugar. Look for statements such as 'no sugar added,' 'unsweetened extra light syrup' or 'juice packed' on the label.
3. Avoid fruits that are canned or frozen in heavy syrup, even if you rinse off the syrup.
4. Drain fruits canned in their own juice. If you drink the drained juice, count it as a separate fruit serving.
5. If you weigh fresh fruit, include the skin, core, seeds and rind.

Exchange List-Meat and Meat Substitutes

Most meats and meat substitutes are good sources of protein. One serving (exchange) of meat or meat substitute usually contains 7 grams of protein. Check the product label to see how much fat and how many calories each product contains.

1. **Lean Meat:** One serving contains 0 to 3 grams of fat and 45 calories. For example, trimmed beef, cheese, fat free cottage cheese, fish, egg whites.
2. **Medium Fat Meat:** One serving contains 4 to 7 grams of fat and 75 calories. For example, beef ground, meat loaf, 3 eggs per week, cheese with 4-7 grams of fat per ounce, fried fish, ricotta cheese.
3. **High Fat Meat:** One serving contains 8 or more grammes of fat and 100 calories. For example, bacon, pork, turkey, regular cheese, sausage and salami.

Exchange List: Milk and Yoghurt

Milk and yoghurt are excellent sources of calcium and protein. One serving (exchange) of milk or yoghurt usually contains 12 grams of carbohydrate and 8 grams of protein. Check the product label to see how much fat and how many calories each product contains.

1. **Fat Free or Low Fat Milk and Yoghurt Products:** One serving contains 0 to 3 grams of fat and 100 calories.

2. **Reduced Fat Milk and Yoghurt Products:** One serving contains 5 grams of fat and 120 calories.

3. **Whole Milk and Yoghurt Products:** One serving contains 8 grams of fat and 160 calories.

Various types of milk and yoghurt may count as slightly different milk and carbohydrate exchanges.

Food Labels

Start With the List of Ingredients

When you are looking at food labels, start with the list of ingredients.

1. **Keep an eye out for heart-healthy ingredients** such as whole wheat flour, soy and oats. Monounsaturated fats such as olive, canola or peanut oils promote heart health too.

2. **Avoid unhealthy ingredients too,** such as hydrogenated or partially hydrogenated oil.

Keep in mind that ingredients are listed in descending order by weight. The main (heaviest) ingredient is listed first, followed by other ingredients used in lesser amounts.

Consider Carbohydrates

If your meal plan is based on carbohydrate counting, food labels become an essential tool for meal planning.

1. **Look at total carbohydrate, not just sugar.** Evaluate the grams of total carbohydrate which includes sugar, complex carbohydrates and fibre, rather than only the grams of sugar. If you zero in on sugar content, you could miss out on nutritious foods naturally high in sugar, such as fruit and milk. And you might overdo foods with no natural or added sugar but plenty of carbohydrate, such as certain cereals and grains.

2. **Don't miss out on high fibre foods.** Pay special attention to high fibre foods. Although the grams of sugar and fibre are counted as part of the grams of total carbohydrate, the count can sometimes be misleading. If a food has 5 grams or more fibre in a serving, the American Diabetes Association recommends subtracting the fibre grams from the total grams of carbohydrate for a more accurate estimate of the product's carbohydrate content.

Sugar Free and Fat Free Products

Always compare the level of carbohydrates in sugar free products with those containing sugar. It is not the calories but the amount of carbohydrates that matter. Same applies to fat free products. They may not be having fat but if the amount of carbs is high, the purpose is still not served.

Know What Counts as a Free Food

A free food is one with:

1. Fewer than 20 calories a serving.
2. Less than 5 grams of carbohydrate a serving.

You can include some free foods in your diet as often as you'd like. Examples include:

1. Diet sodas.
2. Sugar free flavoured gelatin.
3. Sugar free gum.

Diet Tips for Hypertension Control

A key to healthy eating is choosing foods lower in salt and sodium.

Excessive consumption of dietary sodium chloride (salt), coupled with diminished dietary potassium, induces an increase in fluid volume and an impairment of blood pressure regulating mechanisms. This results in hypertension in susceptible individuals.

Most of us consume more salt than we need. NIH recommends limiting the sodium consumption to less than 2.4 grams (2,400 milligrams) of sodium a day. That equals 6 grams (about 1 teaspoon) of table salt a day. The 6 grams include ALL salt and sodium consumed, including that used in cooking and at the table. Recent research has shown that people consuming diets of 1,500 mg of sodium had even better blood pressure lowering benefits. The DASH (dietary approaches to stop hypertension) diet is rich in fruits, vegetables and low fat dairy foods and reduced in total and saturated fat. It is also reduced in red meat, sweets and sugar containing drinks. It is rich in potassium, calcium, magnesium, fibre and protein. Prior studies found that the DASH diet lowers blood pressure and also lowers blood LDL-cholesterol (the 'bad' cholesterol).

Only a small amount of sodium occurs naturally in food items. Most of it is added while processing the food.

Tips to Reduce Salt in Diet

1. Choose fresh food items and not the canned, smoked, or processed variety.
2. Use low sodium salt.
3. Limit intake of pickles, sauces, chutneys, ketchups which have added salt.
4. Avoid having pappad with meals.
5. Do not use flavoured rice, pasta or cereals; they have added salt.
6. Avoid salad dressings and canned soups or curries that are available in the market.
7. Wash the packed or canned food items to remove some of the sodium.
8. Use herbs and other spices instead of salt to make the food palatable and to add flavour to it.
9. Do not eat salty snacks.
10. Do not keep a salt shaker on the dinner table.
11. While eating out, try and have preparations with no MSG (monosodium glutamate).

In order to keep up with the requirement of potassium, a mixed diet consisting of vegetables, fruits, legumes and nuts is recommended.

Chapter 29

Cosmetic Surgery

Well, you may or may not agree with the saying that 'Beauty is only skin deep'. What has happened over the decades is that more and more women have become conscious of their outer beauty. Also cosmetic surgery has become very affordable over the years. We are getting into the habit of going against nature with modern advancements. If a few nips and tucks can enhance your self-esteem and the way you look, a lot us would be willing to go under the knife. There are others from amongst us who feel that nature should be allowed to take its course and one should accept the natural changes which occur with age. But if you are that someone who agrees to go that extra mile to get an image change over there is good news! A number of cosmetic surgery procedures are now available. Cosmetic surgery like any other surgery is associated with a few issues which you need to understand well before hand.

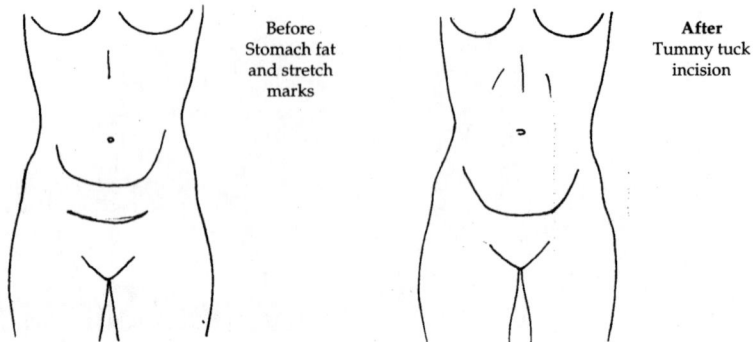

Fig. 29.1: Tummy tuck

Let us become familiar with some of the common cosmetic surgery procedures:

Tummy Tuck

Tummy tuck (abdominoplasty) is a major cosmetic plastic surgery that flattens your abdomen by removing extra fat and skin and tightening muscles in your abdominal wall.

Abdominoplasty is often performed with general anaesthesia. It can also be done using a local anaesthetic with a sedative. There may be some discomfort with local anaesthesia. The tummy tuck surgery takes about 2-5 hours.

Tummy tuck is a major surgical procedure. You can expect a considerable recovery time compared with other plastic surgeries. Most people require 1-3 weeks before returning to work and a normal schedule. Some patients may not need an overnight hospital stay. Others may spend one or two days in the hospital, depending on the extent of the procedure.

Most surgeons recommend that prospective patients kick the cigarette habit for the month before and the month after the tummy tuck. Smoking can cause a delay in wound healing and skin necrosis (death).

After Tummy Tuck Surgery

Your abdomen will be swollen and sore for the first few days. Your surgeon can prescribe pain medication as needed. It is a good idea to exercise after surgery, but only after enough healing time has passed. As a general guideline, tummy tuck patients can start light to moderate activity after 4 weeks. After 6-8 weeks, most people can resume all exercise and activity.

The abdominal scars will appear to worsen during the first 3-6 months. They may take 9 months before they flatten and lighten in colour. People who have had tummy tucks should maintain their result, but they can have a second tummy tuck if they have children again. The good news is that even if you gain and lose a significant amount of weight, you will rarely need a secondary tummy tuck.

Tummy Tuck Risks

1. Anaesthesia risks.
2. Tissue loss.
3. Infection.
4. Collection of blood beneath the skin (haematoma).
5. Collection of fluid under the skim (seroma).
6. Blood clot to the lungs.
7. Aspiration pneumonia.
8. Bleeding under the skin flap.
9. Insufficient healing that may result in the need for a second surgery
10. Death.

Note that these risks are higher in people with underlying medical conditions such as heart or lung disease, poor circulation or diabetes and can be minimised if you follow your surgeon's instructions.

Liposuction

Liposuction is a method of body sculpting, body contouring or 'spot reduction' involving removal of excess, unsightly fat from specific areas of the body. Liposuction can be done in the abdomen, hips, buttocks, back, thighs, knees, calves, ankles, upper arms, jowls, cheeks and neck. It is often done for fat spots which do not respond to exercise.

What to Expect After Liposuction

The suctioned areas will be swollen and uncomfortable for several days after liposuction. In some cases, the small incisions are left open temporarily so that fluids and residual fatty deposits can empty through an inserted drain. Your surgeon may prescribe an antibiotic to reduce the risk of infection.

Usually the treatment area is wrapped with elastic bandage. Support hosiery or a girdle may be worn over this, to help compress tissue and control swelling and bruising. Your surgeon may want you to wear the bandage and/or garment for several days or weeks.

Be patient. The final results may not be evident for up to 6 months, but they are permanent (assuming that your weight remains stable).

Liposuction Risks

All surgeries have risks and liposuction is no exception. They include:

1. Infection.

2. Fluid imbalance. A lot of liquid exists in fat tissue, which is removed during liposuction. What's more, especially during tumescent liposuction, your surgeon may inject large amounts of fluids during liposuction. This can result in a fluid imbalance, which can lead to heart problems, excess fluid collecting in the lungs or kidney problems as your kidneys try to maintain fluid balance.

3. Shock.

4. Blood clots in the lung (pulmonary emboli).

5. Haematoma (a collection of blood in the areas suctioned).

6. Temporary numbness or discolouration in the treated area.

7. Asymmetry, dimpling, wrinkling, unevenness and surface irregularities over the treated area.

8. Perforation wounds in surrounding tissue or organs.

9. Anaesthesia reactions.

10. Swelling.

11. Burns (from ultrasound-assisted and laser-assisted liposuction).

12. Death.

Advantages of Liposuction

Liposuction's advantages include:

1. It is permanent.

2. In competent hands, it has an extremely high safety record.

3. Scars are small and inconspicuous.

Stretch Marks

If you have had a baby or gained a lot of weight, then lost it again, you'll see an unwanted side effect on your physique—stretch marks. Stretch marks, clinically known as striae, are scars left after the dermal and epidermal skin layers lose elasticity due to extreme stretching.

The good news is that stretch marks often fade over time. Those that do not fade can be treated with topical creams and lotions. Exercise is a good way to help prevent stretch marks.

Some people are more genetically susceptible to stretch marks than others. For some, moisturisers and abdominal crunches may not always help. However, for many people there are a variety of treatments that do help.

Treatments

1. **Topical Lotions and Creams:** Many of these products work to firm and tighten the skin. This tightening may lessen the appearance of existing stretch marks by minimising discolouration and depth. Topical Retin-A, hydroxyl creams and products like Stri Vectin-SD tighten skin and temporarily reduce the appearance of stretch marks.

2. **Microdermabrasion and Chemical Peels:** Both these procedures have been used to minimally improve the appearance of scars, reduce discolouration and smooth uneven skin surfaces.

3. **Laser Scar Reduction:** Lasers have recently gained popularity to reduce the colour and depth of stretch marks.

4. **Abdominoplasty:** Some plastic surgeons have noticed stretch mark improvement after an abdominoplasty

procedure. Though, patients are not considered candidates for abdominoplasty for the sole purpose of improving stretch marks. Abdominoplasty is performed to remove excess skin, fat or muscle from the abdomen.

Body Contouring

Body Fat Transfers

For a biocompatible and non-allergenic cosmetic procedure, fat transfers offer a natural way to touch up and round out the edges of small disproportionate body features.

Body Implants

Body implant treatment is a proven method of corrective plastic surgery. Today, a select few plastic surgeons are performing this procedure, which enhances muscular appearance and corrects imbalanced areas of the body.

Body Lift

Whether tightening up after massive weight loss following bariatric surgery (such as Lap Band surgery), or addressing the normal effects of ageing or childbearing, a body lift is an excellent way to contour the abdomen, thighs and buttocks.

Bra-line Back Lift

A new bra-line back lift procedure that removes unsightly back fat rolls while hiding the scar under the bra-line may be the best way to banish sagging skin caused by aging, sun exposure or massive weight loss such as that which occurs after bariatric surgery.

Facelift Variations

There are many types of facelifts.

In general, facelifts differ by:

1. Type of incision.
2. The number of tissue layers treated during the procedure.
3. The area of the face.
4. The degree of invasiveness.

Sometimes facelifts are done in combination with other procedures.

Here you will find basic information on the main types of facelifts, including:

1. SMAS (Superficial Musculoaponeurotic Technique).
2. Deep plane lift.
3. Short scar facelift.
4. Endoscopic facelift.
5. The mid-facelift.
6. Thread lift.
7. Secondary facelift.
8. Combination procedures.

Best Candidates: Anybody aged 45 and up with some neck laxity and some jowling.

Blephroplasty

As we age, excess skin forms in the eye area and the skin loses elasticity. Fatty tissue can accumulate under the skin. Even with good skincare and eyecare, wrinkles, puffiness and drooping eyelids will catch up to you. Plastic surgery may restore a youthful and refreshed appearance to your eyes.

Injectables and Fillers

Cosmetic fillers are not all alike. Injectables and fillers include a variety of materials, like ArteFill, botox, collagen, juviderm, Sculptra which last for different lengths of time and have different effects and uses.

Breast Augmentation

It is one of the favourite procedures of women.

Procedure

Generally, breast enlargement procedure is an outpatient type of surgery that lasts up to two hours. It is important to note that the length of time in surgery is dependent on the type of implant and incision that the patient has decided on. A small incision is made on the breasts and soft silicone implants are inserted. If all things go well during the surgery, the patient is usually sent home on the same day. However, those who encounter problems are advised to stay in the hospital or breast clinic for observation.

Results

Many women leave the hospitals or breast clinics highly satisfied of the results of their breast enlargement procedures. However, there are some breast augmentation procedures that have unsatisfactory results. You must know that implants are to be replaced after a while for varying reasons. It could be due to rupture, aging, weight gain, or loss and the inevitable pull of gravity.

Because breast implant surgery is more often carried out under general anaesthesia it has the same risks as other invasive surgical procedures and in fact any kind of surgical procedure carries a small risk of infection. If the infection cannot be successfully treated with antibiotics, the implant will probably be removed and replaced. The risk of infection is higher if a large haematoma (collection of blood), or seroma (collection of watery fluid) is present immediately after surgery. The body is able to absorb small haematomas or seromas but may need the help of a surgical drain to remove larger ones. Surgical draining can also increase the risk of deflation or rupturing.

It takes a few months for the breasts to settle after breast implant surgery and in this short term patients might experience some swelling, hardness and discomfort with some bruising, twinges and pains possibly over the first few weeks. If patients suffer excessive swelling, deflated breasts, offensive wound discharge or excessive pain or heat in their breast, they should report these symptoms immediately to their surgeon.

Neck-lift

Neck-lift plastic surgery may be performed by a variety of procedures, depending on the individual.

Typically, a neck-lift will include liposuction to remove fat. Cervicoplasty may be included to remove excess skin and platysmaplasty to remove or tighten neck muscles–a process that gets rid of unwanted band lines.

Complications and Risks of Neck-lift

Numbness of the skin occurs often for a few weeks after neck-lift surgery. In rare instances, this condition can be permanent. Other risks include excess scar tissue build up or bruising and puckering of the skin.

As with any plastic surgery, there is a risk of complications related to infection or reaction to anaesthesia. You can avoid most complications by selecting the right plastic surgeon and following pre- and post-operative instructions. With proper precautions by the surgical team, complications are typically minimised or prevented.

Here are some tips to consider when consulting a plastic surgeon:

1. Ask about credentials, type of certification, training and the number of times neck-lifts have been performed in cosmetic surgery practice.
2. View before-and-after photos of patients who received different types of neck-improvement procedures to help set reasonable expectations.
3. Bring a photo to help your doctor see the results you are looking for.
4. Inquire about the type of equipment to be used, where the procedure will be performed and the extent of the procedure.
5. Discuss the possible impact that smoking and existing dental issues may have on your surgery.
6. Review the pre-operative and post-operative instruction list provided by the doctor. These instructions may include:
    i. No eating or drinking after midnight.
    ii. A prescribed antibiotic for before and after the procedure.
    iii. Ceasing certain medications.

Female Hair Loss Treatments

The only FDA-approved medication for female hair loss is the topical solution minoxidil.

This topical solution works on hair follicles to reverse the shrinking process and stimulate new growth on top of the scalp. It is applied twice daily and must be used for at least 4 months to achieve results.

Steroids are often used to treat autoimmune diseases and some doctors are prescribing steroid lotions for women with autoimmune-related hair loss. These steroid-infused lotions can be used with or without minoxidil.

Lasers also play a role in female hair loss treatment. For example, a red light-emitting diode (LED) can stimulate some degree of hair growth by increasing the blood supply to hair follicles that are essentially on life support. In such cases, a laser may help follicles back into a growing stage.

Hair transplants are also increasingly an option for many women. There are many different types of hair transplantation procedures available today to help women achieve a natural look. Hair transplantation involves removing healthy hair follicles from one area of the scalp and transplanting them to the areas of hair loss.

Some women may choose wigs and/or hair weaves to help hide hair loss.

Chapter 30

Alternative Medicine

Let us look at some of the alternative therapies for some of the common health problems of women after the age of 40.

Menopause

Medicinal Herbs

The World Health Organization (WHO) estimates that 4 billion people, 80 per cent of the world population, presently use herbal medicine for some aspect of primary health care. Herbal medicine is a major component in all indigenous peoples' traditional medicine and a common element in ayurvedic, homoeopathic, naturopathic, traditional oriental and native American Indian medicine. WHO notes that of 119 plant-derived pharmaceutical medicines, about 74 per cent are used in modern medicine in ways that correlated directly with their traditional uses as plant medicines by native cultures.

1. **Black cohosh:** Studies of its effectiveness in reducing hot flashes have had mixed results. Recent research suggests that black cohosh does not act like oestrogen,

as once was thought. Black cohosh has had a good safety record over a number of years. Some concerns have been raised about whether it may cause liver problems, but an association has not been proven. Black cohosh is a botanical that is widely available. The most well known brand is Remifemin. The North American Menopause Society reports that black cohosh may be helpful in the very short term (6 months or less) for treatment of hot flashes, night sweats and vaginal dryness. Safety beyond 6 months of use is not known. Side effects are rare and include gastrointestinal upset.

2. **Red clover:** The panel reported that 5 controlled studies found no consistent or conclusive evidence that red clover leaf extract reduces hot flashes. Clinical studies in women report few side effects and no serious health problems have been discussed in the literature. However, there are some cautions. Animal studies have raised concerns that red clover might have harmful effects on hormone sensitive tissue (for example, in the breast and uterus).

3. **Dong quai:** Only one randomised clinical study of dong quai has been done. The researchers did not find it to be useful in reducing hot flashes. Dong quai is known to interact with and increase the activity in the body of, the anti-coagulant drug warfarin. This can lead to bleeding complications in women who take this medicine.

4. **Ginseng:** The panel concluded that ginseng may help with some menopausal symptoms, such as mood symptoms and sleep disturbances and with one's overall sense of well being. However, it has not been found helpful for hot flashes.

5. **Kava:** Kava may decrease anxiety, but there is no evidence that it decreases hot flashes. It is important to note that kava has been associated with liver disease. The FDA has issued a warning to patients and providers about kava because of its potential to damage the liver.

6. **Soy:** The scientific literature includes both positive and negative results for soy extracts on hot flashes. When taken as a food or dietary supplement for short periods of time, soy appears to have few, if any serious side effects. However, long term use of soy extracts has been associated with thickening of the lining of the uterus. Some botanicals, such as phytoestrogens, may help relieve menopause symptoms. Phytoestrogens are substances found in plant-based foods that are thought to have weak oestrogen-like effects. They may work in the body like a weak form of oestrogen. Some may help lower cholestrol levels and have been suggested to relieve hot flashes and night sweats. Examples of plant oestrogens include isoflavones. Isoflavones can be found in foods such as soy products (tofu, soymilk, soybeans).

7. **Evening primrose:** Evening primrose oil is another botanical that is often used to treat hot flashes, although there is no scientific evidence to support this. Side effects include nausea and diarrhoea. Many women with other conditions or those that take certain medications, should not take evening primrose oil.

8. **Flax Seed:** Flax seed is an edible seed that contains lignans, another class of phytoestrogens. Although there is little scientific evidence to support this, flaxseed is thought to decrease the symptoms of menopause, particularly hot flashes. In addition, some studies show that flax seed may lower breast cancer risk in

women. Also known as linseed, flax seed is available in whole seed, ground up meal and seed oil forms. However, only the crushed or ground forms of flax seed contain lignans that your body can digest.

Art Therapies

Art, light and colour therapies go hand in hand. They are all useful in invoking appropriate responses by affecting the mind, body and spirit.

Through art therapy, both adults and children can be helped to express their inner needs and desires and to record the content of dreams and meditations. Art can be a key to the door of the inner mind, externalising thoughts and feelings and thus giving insight into hidden concerns that may be preventing a person from achieving full potential in life.

Art therapies are useful if you have difficulty adjusting emotionally to menopause. It may help you to come to terms creatively and powerfully with this new phase of your life.

Ayurveda

Ayurveda links menopause with aging. Ageing is a Vata (air) stage of life. Thus, the symptoms of menopause experienced by some women are similar to the symptoms seen when the Vata dosha rises and upsets the normal balance of the body. Vata-type menopausal symptoms tend to include depression, anxiety and insomnia. Menopause may also manifest itself in the other two humours. Women with Pitta-type symptoms are often angry and suffer hot flashes. Kapha-type symptoms include listlessness, weight gain and feelings of mental and physical heaviness. The type of treatment depends upon the dosha in which the woman's menopausal symptoms are manifesting.

Treatment for Vata-type Menopause

Excess Vata (air) may be reduced to proper levels by utilising oils, incense, herbs and a special diet.

Sesame, almond and olive oil are among the oils that may be used in massage or placed on specific parts of the body, such as the mouth and ears. Herbs may be mixed with the oils. The vapours from essential oils, such as wintergreen, cinnamon or sandalwood, may be inhaled. Incenses, such as myrrh, frankincense and musk, may also be inhaled.

Treatment for Pitta-type Menopause

Women who display anger and suffer from frequent and severe hot flashes may be suffering from menopausal symptoms associated with excess Pitta (fire). For them, treatment would aim to 'reduce' the Pitta to proper levels. The treatment may utilise oils, incense, herbs and a special diet.

Oils used to combat Pitta-type symptoms include coconut and sesame. You may also take clarified butter, called ghee, internally or use it for massage. In addition, inhaling the vapours from essential oils made from gardenia, honeysuckle, lotus and iris may be recommended, as well as incense made from saffron, jasmine or geraniums.

Herbs to be used include aloe vera, arjuna, barberry, golden seal, gotu kola, motherwort, myrrh, saffron and shatavari. Sandalwood oil is applied to the chest and to the 'third eye'- in the middle of the forehead.

Treatment for Kapha-type Menopause

If the menopause is manifesting in the Kapha (water) humor, the woman may feel unmotivated, tired and bloated. Her treatment would be an anti-Kapha regimen.

Mustard oil and linseed oil are often recommended for this condition. Inhaling the vapours from essential oils made from cedar, pine and sage, as well as incense made from basil, frankincense and cedar, is recommended. The anti-Kapha diet is light, dry and warm.

Acupressure and Acupuncture

Pressure applied to specific points on the hands and feet can help stimulate the ovaries, uterus and adrenal, pituitary, thyroid and parathyroid glands to balance hormone production and reduce hot flashes. Prolonged menstruation can be controlled by applying pressure to the insides of both legs, 5 inches below the knees.

Acupuncture can alleviate many menopausal symptoms by rebalancing the hormonal system, especially headaches and migraines, hot flushing, heavy flooding periods, back pain and sagging skin tone. Heavy and erratic menstrual bleeding in perimenopausal women can be relieved by this technique. Also relieves the pain and headache associated with menstruation.

For Urinary Incontinence

Biofeedback

Several studies report that biofeedback that focuses on the workings of the pelvic floor muscles can help improve bladder control in some women. A transvaginal sensor inserted into the vagina and connected to a computer and monitor measures muscular activity, showing a woman just how effectively she is contracting her pelvic muscles. The monitor presents instant feedback as to which muscles need more training and strengthening.

Once viewed with skepticism, the control of 'involuntary' responses is now seen to be effective in the treatment of migraine headaches, asthma and other disorders in certain individuals.

Diabetes Mellitus

Medicinal Herbs

To date, over 400 traditional plant treatments for diabetes have been reported, although only a small number of these have received scientific and medical evaluation to assess their efficacy. The hypoglycaemic effect of some herbal extracts has been confirmed in human and animal models of type 2 diabetes. The World Health Organization Expert Committee on diabetes has recommended that traditional medicinal herbs be further investigated. The following is a summary of several of the most studied and commonly used medicinal herbs.

Ginseng Species

The root of ginseng has been used for over 2,000 years in the far east for its health promoting properties. Of the several species of ginseng, Panax ginseng (Asian ginseng) and Panax quinquefolius (American ginseng) are commonly used. Constituents of all ginseng species include ginsenosides, polysaccharides, peptides, polyacetylenic alcohol and fatty acids. Most pharmacological actions of ginseng are attributed to ginsenosides, a family of steroids named steroidal saponins. Data from animal studies indicate that both Asian ginseng and American ginseng have significant hypoglycaemic action. This blood glucose-lowering effect appears to be attributed to ginsenoside Rb-2 and more specifically to panaxans I, J, K and L in type 1 diabetic models. But whether these constituents have a similar effect on type 2 diabetes is as yet unknown.

Dietary Supplements and Type 2 Diabetes

Some people with diabetes use CAM therapies for their health condition. For example, they may try accupuncture or biofeedback to help with painful symptoms. Some use dietary supplements in efforts to improve their blood glucose control, manage symptoms and lessen the risk of developing serious complications such as heart problems.

ALA (ALPHA LIPOIC ACID) has been researched for its effect on insulin sensitivity, glucose metabolism and diabetic neuropathy. Some studies have found benefits, but more research is needed. (There are some studies, reported from outside the United States, of ALA delivered intravenously; however, this research is outside the scope of this fact sheet.)

Because ALA might lower blood sugar too much, people with diabetes who take it must monitor their blood sugar levels very carefully.

Chromium is an essential trace mineral that is, the body requires small amounts of it to function properly. Some people with diabetes take chromium in an effort to improve their blood glucose control. Chromium is found in many foods, but usually only in small amounts; relatively good sources include meat, whole grain products and some fruits, vegetables and spices. In supplement form (capsules and tablets), it is sold as chromium picolinate, chromium chloride and chromium nicotinate.

Chromium supplementation has been researched for its effect on glucose control in people with diabetes. Study results have been mixed. Some researchers have found benefits, but many of the studies have not been well designed. Additional, high quality research is needed.

At low doses, short term use of chromium appears to be safe for most adults. However, people with diabetes should be aware that chromium might cause blood sugar levels to go too low. High doses can cause serious side effects, including kidney problems—an issue of special concern to people with diabetes.

Omega-3 fatty acids are polyunsaturated fatty acids that come from foods such as fish, fish oil, vegetable oil (primarily canola and soybean), walnuts and wheat germ. Omega-3 supplements are available as capsules or oils (such as fish oil). Omega-3's are important in a number of bodily functions, including the movement of calcium and other substances in and out of cells, the relaxation and contraction of muscles, blood clotting, digestion, fertility, cell division and growth. In addition, omega-3's are thought to protect against heart disease, reduce inflammation and lower triglyceride levels.

Omega-3 fatty acids have been researched for their effect on controlling glucose and reducing heart disease risk in people with type 2 diabetes. Studies show that omega-3 fatty acids lower triglycerides, but do not affect blood glucose control, total cholesterol or HDL (good) cholesterol in people with diabetes. In some studies, omega-3 fatty acids also raised LDL (bad) cholesterol. Additional research, particularly long term studies that look specifically at heart disease in people with diabetes, is needed.

Omega-3's appear to be safe for most adults at low-to-moderate doses. Safety questions have been raised about fish oil supplements, because some species of fish can be contaminated by substances such as mercury, pesticides or PCBs (Polychlorinated biphenyl). In high doses, fish oil can interact with certain medications, including blood thinners and drugs used for high blood pressure.

Polyphenols—antioxidants found in tea and dark chocolate, among other dietary sources—are being studied for possible effects on vascular health (including blood pressure) and on the body's ability to use insulin.

Laboratory studies suggest that EGCG (Epigallocatechin gallate), a polyphenol found in green tea, may protect against cardiovascular disease and have a beneficial effect on insulin activity and glucose control. However, a few small clinical trials studying EGCG and green tea in people with diabetes have not shown such effects.

No adverse effects of EGCG (Epigallocatechin gallate) or green tea were discussed in these studies. Green tea is safe for most adults when used in moderate amounts. However, green tea contains caffeine, which can cause, in some people, insomnia, anxiety or irritability, among other effects. Green tea also has small amounts of vitamin K, which can make anticoagulant drugs, such as warfarin, less effective.

Hypercholesterolemia

Herbal/nutritional supplements that might help lower cholesterol:

Garlic: According to some studies, garlic might decrease blood levels of total cholesterol by a few percentage points. Other studies, however, suggest that it might not be as beneficial as once thought. It might also have significant side effects and/or interactions with certain medicines. Garlic might prolong bleeding and blood clotting time, so garlic and garlic supplements should not be consumed prior to surgery and should not be taken with blood thinning medicines such as warfarin (brand name Coumadin).

Guggulipid: Guggulipid is the gum resin of the mukul myrrh tree. In clinical studies performed in India, guggulipid significantly reduced blood levels of total cholesterol, LDL-C and triglycerides.

Other Herbal Products

The results of several studies suggest the cholesterol-lowering action of the following:

1. Fenugreek seeds and leaves.
2. Artichoke leaf extract.
3. Yarrow.
4. Holy basil.

These and other commonly used herbs and spices—including ginger, turmeric and rosemary—are being investigated for their potential beneficial effects relating to coronary disease prevention. These products appear to have anti-inflammatory properties.

Chronic inflammation has been recently recognized as an important factor in the development and progression of coronary heart disease and cancer. These herbs/spices are extensively used in traditional culinary practices and are considered safe. Even without the strong evidence for their cholesterol-lowering actions, these herbs can add extra flavour and nutritional value to plant-based diets that should be at the center of efforts to reduce blood cholesterol levels and decrease the risk of coronary heart disease.

Dietary Elements that Aid in Lowering Cholesterol

Increased consumption of dietary fibre soy foods and plant compounds similar to cholesterol (plant stanols and sterols) can significantly reduce blood levels of LDL-C, or 'bad' cholesterol.

Fibre

Only plant foods contain dietary fibre.

These include:

1. Vegetables.
2. Fruits.
3. Legumes.
4. Unrefined grains.

The soluble fibre found in foods such as oat bran, psyllium seeds, apples and citrus fruits are particularly effective in reducing increased cholesterol. The FDA now allows the claim on food packaging that diets rich in whole grains and other plant foods and low in saturated fat and cholesterol, might help reduce the risk of heart disease.

Soybeans

Soybeans have been shown to reduce the risk of coronary heart disease development by acting on LDL-C in three ways:

1. Decreasing LDL-C blood levels.
2. Increasing the size of LDL-C particles.
3. Preventing the particles' oxidation (the process whereby LDL particles are chemically changed by oxygen and more likely to damage blood vessels).

Dietary soybean proteins decrease blood levels of not only LDL-C, but also of triglycerides, another type of fat that can increase the risk of heart disease. Soy protein is present in tofu, tempeh, soy milk, soy, yoghurt and many other food products made from soybeans. FDA has approved the health claim on packaged foods that the inclusion of soy protein foods in a diet low in saturated fat and cholesterol promotes heart health.

Phytosterols

Phytosterols (plant sterol and stanol esters) are compounds found in whole grains as well as in many vegetables, fruits and vegetable oils. They decrease blood LDL-C, mostly by interfering with the intestinal absorption of cholesterol. FDA allows the use of health claims that link plant sterol/stanol esters and a reduced risk of coronary heart disease on the labeling of certain products that contain these phytosterols.

The Benefits of these Dietary Elements

Dietary fibre, soybeans and phytosterols decrease blood cholesterol levels by different mechanisms. Therefore, it is not surprising that the combined dietary intake of these foods and other plant substances, along with a low intake of saturated fats, is more effective at reducing cholesterol levels than each individual substance alone.

Though dietary intervention should be the primary step in an effort to reduce elevated cholesterol levels, often recommended reduced fat diets might not contain enough plant foods and still include too much meat and too high a level of saturated fat to be effective at lowering cholesterol to truly effective levels.

If a plant-based diet alone is not effective at reducing cholesterol levels to truly effective levels, such a diet should be combined with cholesterol-lowering medicines. Recent reports provide support for an impressive effectiveness of such an approach compared to a standard, reduced fat diet in combination with cholesterol-lowering drugs.

Low fat, plant-based diets have many benefits that go beyond cholesterol reduction. Such diets help in the prevention, arrest or even reversal of coronary heart disease. In addition, there is a growing body of evidence that such diets also might reduce the risk of several common types of cancer, high blood pressure, diabetes and obesity.

Uterine Fibroids

Fibroid growths in the uterus can cause infertility, pain, urinary incontinence and heavy bleeding. Traditional Chinese herbal medicine reduces fibroids in many cases.

An alternative to hormone therapy or surgery, traditional Chinese herbal medicine offers safe options for reducing fibroid masses in the uterus. For many women these centuries old treatments are regaining popularity.

Traditional Chinese Herbal Treatment of Fibroids

In traditional Chinese medicine, Yin Deficiency Fire, Liver Qi Stagnation with Spleen Qi Deficiency or Qi and Blood Stagnation are the three ways in which fibroids might present themselves to the TCM practitioner. Thus in Chinese medicine, there are three very different approaches to treating uterine fibroid masses depending on the individual woman's signs and symptoms.

Yin deficiency fire is common in women who use up their yin or feminine energy over time. Chronic illness may also result in yin deficiency. In this case, a formula which drains the fire while supporting the yin would be used. American ginseng might be included in this case.

Qi stagnation is often brought on by emotional stress. Both qi stagnation and blood stasis may be a result of trauma as in major surgery, a significant injury or even a difficult childbirth. When the blood and qi are blocked from moving smoothly around the body aches, pains and masses often result. Dong quai and other herbs may be used in a formula to both invigorate and tonify qi and blood is appropriate for women presenting with qi and blood stagnation.

Spleen qi deficiency with Liver qi stagnation is the third way in which fibroids may present in traditional

Chinese medicine. Women with this pattern may present with digestive problems and irritability. The formula used for these women might include hawthrn fruits (Shan zha).

Several alternative therapies offer ways to reduce oestrogen levels naturally. The hope is to forestall or eliminate the need for a hysterectomy.

Mind/Body Medicine for Uterine Fibroids

For women with fibroids, mind/body medicine focuses on significantly reducing stress. This is vital because stress can interrupt the development and release of eggs (a process called ovulation). When this process does not happen, the body's level of oestrogen remains unnecessarily high, precipitating fibroid development. Mind/body medicine offers many therapies that teach relaxation and how to lower stress levels, including:

1. Forms of guided imagery and creative visualisation.
2. Meditation.
3. Yoga (including breathing exercises and stretches).
4. Biofeedback.
5. Dance therapy.
6. Hypnotherapy.
7. Spirituality.

Here's an example of a relaxation breathing exercise that would be part of a guided imagery regimen:

1. Wearing loose clothing, lie down or sit in a comfortable chair.
2. Slowly close your eyes. Begin breathing deeply and slowly.
3. When exhaling, imagine tension effortlessly flowing out of your body with each breath.

4. As you inhale, picture yourself filling your body with fresh air and energy.

5. Continue the slow, deep breathing for as long as you are comfortable.

Hydrotherapy for Uterine Fibroids

Hydrotherapy directed at the lower abdomen can stimulate blood circulation, which delivers nutrients and other beneficial substances to the cells and cleans away waste products. These treatments can also provide pain relief. Castor oil, made from the leaves of the castor oil plant, is commonly applied to the lower abdomen as a warm pack.

The cold-pressed oil contains a substance that boosts the action of cells important to the immune system. Alternating hot and cold sitz baths can also be effective.

Nutritional Therapy for Uterine Fibroids

According to nutritional therapy, diet and supplements can stabilize or even lower the levels of oestrogen in the body. As oestrogen amounts drop, existing fibroids should shrink and new ones can be prevented. Diet and supplements may also reduce some of the symptoms of fibroids.

One of liver's roles in the body is to break down oestrogens. Therefore, the diet should allow the liver to do its work and not include foods that can tax this organ. These taxing foods to be avoided include:

1. Sugar.
2. Meat.
3. Dairy products.
4. Alcohol.

In addition, meat and dairy products can be a source of hormones (including oestrogen) from livestock. Because they are also high in fat and oestrogen is stored in fat cells, these foods may cause additional problems for women with fibroids. Instead, focus on eating fresh vegetables and fruits, whole grains, nuts and raw seeds. These steps should also result in a diet that's high in fibre and low in fat.

The B vitamins also aid the liver and are recommended. They can be added in the form of whole foods (such as lentils, rice bran and blackstrap molasses), or supplements. Vitamin B6, in particular, enhances the breakdown and removal of oestrogen from the body.

Natural plant oestrogens, called phytoestrogens, can actually compete with human oestrogen in the body, resulting in an overall lower level of oestrogen. Soybeans are a good food source of this substance and can be used as a whole cooked bean or in its other forms, including tofu, tempeh and soy milk.

Researchers have linked heavy menstrual bleeding with low levels of vitamin A in the blood. One study gave women doses of vitamin A for 15 days, after which time menstrual bleeding was reduced in about 90 per cent of the patients. To achieve proper levels of vitamin A in the body, most practitioners of nutritional therapy recommend eating foods rich in beta-carotene (such as carrots and sweet potatoes) or taking beta-carotene supplements. A naturopathic physician may recommend a programme of several supplements to normalize oestrogen levels, including B vitamins; vitamin E; beta-carotene; cysteine, methionine, choline, inositol (to help the liver metabolize oestrogen and other substances more efficiently); and iron (if the fibroids cause heavy menstrual bleeding and anaemia). Dietary recommendations include adopting a low fat, high fibre diet and avoiding meat, dairy products, eggs, refined sugar and caffeine.

Other Therapies for Uterine Fibroids

1. **Acupressure for Uterine Fibroids**: Points along the liver and spleen channels are often targeted for symptom relief.

2. **Herbal Medicine for Uterine Fibroids**: Some herbs that can ease the symptoms of fibroids are blue cohosh, dong quai and wild cherry.

3. **Homoeopathy for Uterine Fibroids**: Remedies for short term relief of symptoms can be very effective, but a careful diagnosis by a professional is necessary to tailor a long term remedy for fibroids.

4. **Detoxification, Fasting and Colon Therapy for Uterine Fibroids**: Several types of treatments can remove toxins and prevent certain organs (such as the liver) from being overworked. These therapies can also alleviate constipation and haemorrhoids related to fibroids.

Dysfunctional Uterine Bleeding

The results of meta-analysis of clinical practice demonstrated that CHM used under the guidelines of basic TCM theory gained encouraging results in the treatment of DUB (dysfunctional uterine bleeding), especially when combined with western medicine. Most women in the included trials stopped bleeding and many of them regained normal menstruation in a certain period of time. No adverse events were reported due to (in part) the use of herbs which are mostly not noxious with few side effects. A great deal of emphasis was placed on treatment based on differentiation. Modification of corresponding assistant and adjunctive herbs in formulas according to the accompanying symptoms is very common in these studies. Lumping trials of herbal compounds with the same or similar effects together had not caused heterogeneity, which, perhaps, is a prospective method for TCM formulas varying widely in constituents when performing meta-analysis.

Due to the lack of trials comparing CHM with no treatment or placebo, it is impossible to evaluate the effectiveness of CHM. CHM treatment in these studies seems to show a favourable comparative effect on the control of western **medicine**. However, the poor methodological quality may weaken the validity of the results. Owing to the lack of RCTs with high methodologic quality, we have to wait. In this case, the waiting period could be a time to develop hypotheses to explain the results that have been achieved in individuals and trials conducted lower on the golden pyramid. Per**for**ming clinical trials with high methodological quality of TCM **for DUB** is very helpful to accurately assess the benefits and potential risks in the treatment of **DUB**. In the future, more rigorously designed, randomized, double-blind, placebo-controlled trials with large sample sizes are needed to make TCM accepted by more people in the world.

Heart Disease

According to Bolling, surveys indicate that between 60 per cent and 70 per cent of people with cardiovascular disease use CAM. The problem is that there can be just as many drug-herb interactions as there are drug-drug interactions, he says.

Bolling says some people take dandelion, dandelion wine or dandelion extract for hypertension. The herb reputedly works as a diuretic and results in potassium loss. However, as with many herbal supplements, reliable scientific data are scarce. If a patient taking a prescribed diuretic also takes dandelion, potassium loss could be exacerbated and raise the risk for cardiac arrhythmia.

Some people take yohimbine, an alpha dilator that is extracted from the bark of an African tree, for erectile dysfunction. If a person takes too much or is taking an anti-depressant, Bolling says, yohimbine could trigger a hypertensive crisis.

Vogel says that blue cohosh, used for muscle stimulation and stimulation of labour, blocks the effect of some blood pressure medications.

Bearberry is used as a diuretic and increases the effect of digoxin, which many patients take to increase heart muscle activity. The danger, Vogel says, is that this herb can deplete potassium and cause toxicity of the heart medication.

Even physicians who have taken time to learn about complementary therapies say there is not yet enough evidence to endorse their use. But some physicians say they do not discourage patients from biofeedback, meditation, acupuncture and other therapies that might decrease stress levels and have not been shown to cause any harm.

'Both meditation and acupuncture have shown some promise in the short term improvement of blood pressure,' says Daniel Jones, MD, of the University of Mississippi Medical Center. "Most of the studies that are being done are not very well controlled and almost all of them are short term studies. Of course, there are many things that will modulate blood pressure for the short term that do not appear to have a long term impact on blood pressure. That's part of the challenge in this area of study."

The evidence is "not strong enough, at this point, for any alternative therapies," Jones says.

The biggest risk of a physician recommending complementary or alternative therapies is that the patient might use them in lieu of blood pressure medications, experts say.

Studies have suggested, that fish oil, or omega-3 fatty acids, might have a fair effect on systolic blood pressure, lowering it by about 3 mm of Hg.

There is conflicting evidence, but some studies indicate a modest effect on blood pressure from mind-body interventions, including biofeedback, behavioural modification, meditation, breathing exercises, guided imagery and more. This effect can range from a 3 to a 5 mm of Hg drop in systolic blood pressure, depending on the study'.

In general, there is little evidence to warrant a physician recommending any CAM (Complimentary and Alternative Medicine) therapy, except for diet (which is considered a main stream treatment). Doctors need to stress upon the importance of lifestyle changes and medications so that people do not misconstrue a physician's support of an alternative therapy as a recommended alternative to conventional treatment.

Depression

The only true stand-alone CAM therapy for depression is St. John's wort. All other CAM therapies are typically considered adjuncts (additions) to other treatments. The following therapies are currently being studied to determine whether they benefit people with depression. These therapies are generally not harmful, but it is unclear whether they are truly helpful. There is some limited research on the effectiveness of these therapies, but study results do not allow us to suggest them as stand-alone treatments for depression.

B Vitamins

B vitamins, especially B1 (thiamine), B6 (pyridoxine), B9 (folic acid) and B12 (cobalamin) have all been examined for their contribution to depression. These B vitamins play many important roles in the body and are necessary to manufacture brain chemicals (GABA, serotonin, dopamine and others) responsible for regulating the mood.

Many studies on effectiveness of using B vitamins for treating depression are promising. However, many more studies must be conducted before concluding that these vitamins are effective in treating all types of depression. Research suggests that the B vitamins tend to work well for depression related to a deficiency state (such as with alcoholics or other people with poor nutrition), or for depression associated with premenstrual syndrome.

B vitamins enhance the effects of many of the standard treatments for depression. Trials of standard anti-depressant medications combined with B vitamins indicated that people recover from depression more rapidly and often with fewer side effects when taking this combination.

The B vitamins are water-soluble (dissolvable in water) and are easily removed from the body in the urine. They are generally considered safe, with little to no side effects. However, mega doses (very high doses) of B6 (pyridoxine) have been associated with liver inflammation and nerve damage. It is best to take a multivitamin that contains many B vitamins (such as a multi-B vitamin combination), or a separate B complex supplement. Follow the dosing instructions on the vitamin label or consult with your health care practitioner.

Homoeopathy

The mechanisms by which homoeopathy achieves treatment effects is unclear. Many scientists suggest that when homoeopathy works, benefits are caused by the so-called placebo effect (patients taking inactive medications show symptom improvement because they think they are receiving active drugs). This has not been established definitively, however. Some clinical trials have shown that homoeopathy works better than a placebo (medication without an active ingredient) for treating depression, but other studies have not shown this result. In any event, most homoeopathic preparations are so diluted that there is very little chance that an active ingredient (in the conventional sense) is present.

While there are many self-help books on homoeopathy, it is best to go to a practitioner and have them personalize a remedy for you. Because homoeopathy uses such small amounts of substances, it can be said that homoeopathy has no side effects or drug interactions.

Yoga

Similar to exercise, yoga has shown some promise as a treatment for depression. Many yoga practices incorporate deep breathing, stretching and strengthening exercises along with a mild cardiovascular workout in a class atmosphere.

Yoga is difficult to study in a clinical setting because there are several different factors that can impact its effectiveness. For example, there are many different types of yoga (with varied levels of relaxation or activity) and individual levels of effort during classes may vary. In addition, only certain people are willing to try this form of exercise, so study results may not apply to every group of people who are depressed. There are a few studies that suggest that regular yoga sessions improve depressive symptoms, but their design makes it difficult to draw broad conclusions about the type of person who would benefit most from this therapy.

Yoga can be practiced at home, or you can find a class at a local community/recreation center, gym, or yoga studio. There are forms of yoga that incorporate slow stretching and others that are more active. If you are thinking of trying yoga, visit a class a few times to determine which teacher and style will best meet your needs.

Acupuncture

Acupuncture literally means 'needle piercing' and is the practice of inserting very fine needles into the skin to stimulate specific anatomic (body) points for therapeutic purposes. In addition to needles, acupuncturists can also use heat, pressure, friction, suction or electromagnetic energy impulses to stimulate acupuncture points. Treatment is designed to balance the movement of energy (called qi) in the body to restore health.

Acupuncture has shown some promise as a treatment for depression. Once again, the varied treatments (how the needles are used) and selection bias (only certain types of people are willing to try acupuncture) affect research trials, making it difficult to determine if acupuncture is helpful for all types of people with depression. Further study is required.

The specific course and duration of acupuncture treatment depends on the nature and severity of depressive symptoms. A typical course of treatment might involve 10-12 weekly sessions.

Osteoarthritis

Acupuncture

During acupuncture, tiny needles are inserted into your skin at precise spots. Practitioners believe the needles free or redirect your body's energy in order to relieve pain. Studies of acupuncture for knee osteoarthritis have been mixed. Most studies haven't found a benefit, though some have found some short term relief of pain. Acupuncture can be safe if you select a reputable practitioner—ask your doctor to suggest someone. Risks include infection, bruising and some pain where needles are inserted into your skin.

Ginger

The ginger plant is best known for its use in cooking, but some research has found that the ginger extract may be helpful in reducing osteoarthritis pain. Limited studies have been conducted with ginger in people with osteoarthritis and results have been mixed. Side effects of ginger supplements can include heartburn and diarrhoea. It may interfere with warfarin.

Glucosamine and Chondroitin

Studies have been mixed on these nutritional supplements. Some have found benefits for people with osteoarthritis, while others haven't. Tell your doctor if you are considering taking these supplements. Do not use glucosamine if you are allergic to shellfish.

Magnets

Some people believe placing magnets near your affected joint can relieve osteoarthritis pain. Some small studies have found magnets can provide temporary pain relief, though others haven't found any benefit from magnets. It isn't clear how magnet therapy might work. Still, a variety of magnetic products, such as bracelets are available. Magnets appear to be safe.

Tai Chi and Yoga

These movement therapies involve gentle exercises and stretches combined with deep breathing. Many people use these therapies to abate stress in their lives, though small studies have found that tai chi and yoga may reduce osteoarthritis pain. More study is needed to understand whether tai chi and yoga can relieve osteoarthritis pain. Talk to your doctor if you would like to give tai chi or yoga a try. When led by a knowledgeable instructor, these therapies are safe. But do not do any moves that cause pain in your joints.

Urinary Tract Infection

Herbs

Herbs may be used as dried extracts (capsules, powders, teas), glycerites (glycerine extracts), or tinctures (alcohol extracts). Teas should be made with 1 teaspoon herb per cup of hot water. Steep covered 5-10 minutes for leaf or flowers and 10-20 minutes for roots.

Start herbal therapy at the first sign of symptoms and continue for 3 days after you start feeling better. Teas work best for treating UTIs because the additional fluid intake helps the 'flushing action'. Combine 2 herbs from each of the following categories and drink 4-6 cups per day.

Urinary Antiseptics are Antimicrobial: Uva ursi (Arctostaphylos uva ursi), buchu (Agathosma betulina), thyme leaf (Thymus vulgaris), pipissewa (Chimaphila umbellata).

Urinary Astringents Tone and Heal the Urinary Tract: Horsetail (Equisetum arvense), plantain (Plantago major).

Urinary Demulcents Soothe the Inflamed Urinary Tract: Corn silk (Zea maydis), couch grass (Agropyron repens).

Marshmallow root (Althaea officinalis) is best used alone in a cold infusion. Soak 1 heaped teaspoon of marshmallow root in 1 quart of cold water overnight. Strain and drink during the day in addition to any other urinary tea.

For advanced or recurrent infections prepare a tincture of equal parts of golden seal (Hydrastis canadensis) and cone flower (Echinacea purpurea). Take 30 drops, 4-6 times per day.

Homoeopathy

There have been few studies examining the effectiveness of specific homoeopathic remedies. Professional homoeopaths, however, may recommend one or more of the following treatments for UTI based on their knowledge and clinical experience. Before prescribing a remedy, homoeopaths take into account a person's constitutional type. In homoeopathic terms, a person's constitution is his or her physical, emotional and intellectual make up. An experienced homoeopath assesses all of these factors when determining the most appropriate remedy for a particular individual.

Apis mellifica: For stinging or burning pains that tend to worsen at night and from warmth; individuals for whom this remedy is appropriate feel an intense urge to urinate, yet can only do so in drops.

Aconitum napellus: For early symptoms of UTI, particularly with extremely painful urination that is often described as a hot sensation.

Berberis vulgaris: For UTIs with burning or shooting pains during urination that may radiate to the pelvis and/

or back; when not urinating, an aching sensation is present in the bladder that worsens with movement; pains may also extend to legs and abdomen.

Cantharis vesicatoria: This is the most common and considered the most effective homoeopathic remedy for UTI; this remedy is most appropriate for individuals who are restless, experience a burning sensation, have decreased urine flow (despite a strong desire to urinate) and have increased sexual desire despite symptoms.

Mercurius vivus: For burning urination and a strong urge to urinate; symptoms worsen at night and tend to be accompanied by chills and sweating; urine is dark and only small amounts pass; burning sensation is often worse when the individual is not urinating.

Nux vomica: For individuals who have a constant urge to urinate; pain is described as needle-like; urge to have a bowel movement may accompany urinary urgency; mild, temporary relief may be experienced from urination and warm baths; symptoms may begin following ingestion of alcohol, coffee, drugs, or overeating.

Pulsatilla pratensis: For bladder inflammation that begins after an individual develops a sudden chill in hot weather; this remedy is most appropriate for individuals with an urgent desire to urinate who may be emotional, crave attention and dribble urine after laughing, coughing, sneezing or being surprised.

Sarsaparilla officinalis: For women who experience severe pain at the end of urination and who, occasionally, may feel compelled to stand to urinate.

Staphysagria: For UTIs usually associated with sexual intercourse or following extreme embarrassment or humiliation, particularly from sexual abuse; this remedy is most appropriate for those who have an urgent desire to urinate and have the sensation that a single drop of urine is still present even following urination.

Osteoporosis

Acupuncture

Acupuncture can increase energy, improve mood and reduce pain, making it possible to get back into motion and therefore indirectly help to protect your bones. Biofeedback and relaxation techniques, such as meditation, can also achieve these results by reducing stress, which may enable you to participate in more physical activity.

Diet

Eating an osteporosis-friendly diet is recommended as part of an osteoporosis management plan. In addition to reviewing your intake of calcium, vitamin D and other vitamins and minerals, a CAM physician will make recommendations about other elements of your diet and may suggest specific foods to incorporate. As an example, 1 review of existing data from 17 clinical trials concluded that isoflavones from soy or red clover may help strengthen women's bones after menopause.

Herbs

Traditional Chinese herbal practitioners may suggest herbal teas, soups and other therapies that can affect calcium use by your body. For your own safety, just be sure to work with a Chinese herbal practitioner who is certified by the National Certification Commission for Acupuncture and Oriental Medicine (NCCAOM).

Nutritional Supplements

You might consider using a bone-building supplement that includes calcium, zinc, magnesium, boron and the other vitamins and minerals necessary for healthy bones, according to Frye.

Not all CAM treatments are created equal, warns Frye, who cautions against using yam cream, a heavily promoted natural cream produced from wild yams. 'We call it the yam scam because it has no real effect,' she says. Yam cream contains the active ingredient diosgenin, which promoters say can be converted to female hormones within the human body and therefore protect against osteoporosis. But there is no good evidence to support this, nor is there any evidence to support the use of progesterone creams.

If you are considering CAM treatments, make sure you keep your primary doctor in the loop to avoid any interference between the CAM therapy and your regular osteoporosis treatment. Another word of caution: People with osteoporosis and fractures must also be realistic about what these treatments can achieve—CAM therapies may help strengthen bones (research is ongoing), but they cannot cure osteoporosis.

Stress

Meditation Techniques

This meditation process is good to induce a relaxation response. Plan to make meditation a regular part of your daily routine. Set aside 10-20 minutes each day at the same time, if possible. Before breakfast is a good time.

Choose a quiet spot where you will not be disturbed by other people or by the telephone.

Procedure

1. Sit quietly in a comfortable position. Refer to the section on postures for recommendations on sitting positions.
2. Eliminate distractions and interruptions during the period you'll be meditating.
3. Commit yourself to a specific length of time and try to stick to it.
4. Pick a focus word or short phrase that's firmly rooted in your personal belief system. A non-religious person might choose a neutral word like one, peace or love. Others might use the opening words of a favourite prayer from their religion such as 'Hail Mary full of Grace', 'I surrender all to you', 'Hallelujah', 'Om', etc.
5. Close your eyes. This makes it easy to concentrate.
6. Relax your muscles sequentially from head to feet. This helps to break the connection between stressful thoughts and a tense body. Starting with your forehead, become aware of tension as you breathe in. Let go of any obvious tension as you breathe out. Go through the rest of your body in this way, proceeding down through your eyes, jaws, neck, shoulders, arms, hands, chest, upper back, middle back and midriff, lower back, belly, pelvis, buttocks, thighs, calves and feet.
7. Breathe slowly and naturally, repeating your focus word or phrase silently as you exhale.
8. Assume a passive attitude. Do not worry about how well you are doing. When other thoughts come to mind, simply say, 'Oh, well,' and gently return to the repetition.
9. Continue for 10-20 minutes. You may open your eyes to check the time, but do not use an alarm.

10. After you finish, sit quietly for a minute or so, at first with your eyes closed and later with your eyes open. Do not stand for one or two minutes.

11. Plan for a session once or twice a day.

Health Conditions That are Benefited by Meditation

1. Drug Addiction

The transcendental meditation technique has proven to be a successful coping strategy in helping to deal with drug addiction, a useful tool in psycho-neuro-immunology (PNI) by helping control the immune system and an effective manager of stress and pain.

2. Prolonging Life Expectancy

A strong link has also been established between the practice of TM and longevity. Only two factors have been scientifically determined to actually extend life–caloric restriction and lowering of the body's core temperature. Meditation has been shown to lower core body temperature.

3. Stress Control

Most of the people who get on meditation do so because of its beneficial effects on stress. Stress refers to any or all the various pressures experienced in life. These can stem from work, family, illness or environment and can contribute to such conditions as anxiety, hypertension and heart disease. How an individual sees things and how he or she handles them makes a big difference in terms of how much stress he or she experiences.

Research has shown that hormones and other biochemical compounds in the blood indicative of stress tend to decrease during transcendental meditation practice. These changes also stabilize over time, so that a person is actually less stressed biochemically during daily activity.

This reduction of stress translates directly into a reduction of anxiety and tension. Literally dozens of studies have shown this.

4. Pain Management

Chronic pain can systematically erode the quality of life. Although great strides are being made in traditional medicine to treat recurring pain, treatment is rarely as simple as prescribing medication or surgery.

Anxiety decreases the threshold for pain and pain causes anxiety. The result is a vicious cycle. Compared with people who feel relaxed, those under stress experience pain more intensely and become even more stressed, which aggravates their pain. Meditation breaks this cycle.

Childbirth preparation classes routinely teach pregnant women deep breathing exercises to minimize the pain and anxiety of labour. Few call it breath meditation, but that's what it is.

Meditative techniques are also a key element in the arthritis self-help course at Stanford University. More than 100,000 people with arthritis have taken the 12 hour course and learned meditation-style relaxation exercises as part of a comprehensive self-care programme. Graduates report a 15 to 20 per cent reduction in pain.

In one study overseen by Dr Kabat-Zinn, 72 per cent of the patients with chronic pain conditions achieved at least a 33 per cent reduction after participating in an 8 week period of mindful meditation, while 61 per cent of the pain patients achieved at least a 50 per cent reduction. Additionally, these people perceived their bodies as being 30 per cent less problematic, suggesting an overall improvement in self-esteem and positive views regarding their bodies.

Meditation may not eliminate pain, but it helps people cope more effectively.

5. Cancer and Other Chronic Illness

Meditation and other approaches to deep relaxation help center people so they can figure out how they'd like to handle the illness and proceed with life. Dr Ainslie Meares, an Australian psychiatrist who uses meditation with cancer patients, studied 73 patients who had attended at least 20 sessions of intensive meditation and wrote: 'Nearly all such patients can expect significant reduction of anxiety and depression, together with much less discomfort and pain. There is reason to expect a 10 per cent chance of quite remarkable slowing of the rate of growth of the tumour and a 50 per cent chance of greatly improved quality of life'.

6. Heart Disease

Meditation is a key component of Ornish therapy, the only treatment scientifically proven to reverse heart disease.

7. High Blood Pressure

As soon as Dr Benson learned that transcendental meditation reliably reduced blood pressure in meditators, he taught the relaxation response to 36 people with moderately elevated blood pressure. After several weeks of practice, their average blood pressure declined significantly, reducing their risk of stroke and heart attack.

8. Infertility

Couples dealing with infertility may become depressed, anxious and angry. To help them cope, Alice D. Domar, PhD, a psychologist at the Mind/Body Medical Institute, taught the relaxation response to one group of infertile couples. Compared with a similar group of infertile couples who did not learn deep relaxation, the meditators experienced less distress and were more likely to get pregnant.

9. Premenstrual Syndrome (PMS), Tension Headaches

Meditation can ease physical complaints such as premenstrual syndrome (PMS), tension headaches and other common health problems.

Meditation gives people a psychological buffer so that life's hectic pace does not knock them out. Practicing meditation is like taking a vacation once or twice a day. When you nurture yourself, you accrue tremendous spin-off benefits.

For example, when you are under high stress, it can worsen symptoms of PMS because stress can cause the muscle tension associated with PMS complaints such as fatigue, soreness and aching. On the other hand, when you meditate regularly, you dramatically reduce your body's response to stress and that can ease the discomfort associated with PMS. The results may not be apparent for several months. You will probably need to meditate regularly for several months before your body responds positively.

10. Irritable Bowel Syndrome, Ulcers and Insomnia

Meditation can also improve irritable bowel syndrome, ulcers and insomnia, among other stress related conditions. 80 per cent of the people who use meditation to relieve insomnia are successful.

Meditation can help prevent or treat stress related complaints such as anxiety, headaches and bone, muscle and joint problems. Meditation also provides an inner sense of clarity and calm and that, in itself, may help ward off certain illnesses.

Chapter 31

Screening Tests for Women Over 40 Years

As women age, their chances of suffering from diseases increase. However, if detected early, many diseases, including many early stages of cancer, can be treated successfully. For this, certain screening tests should be undertaken by all the women after the age of 40 as per recommendations or requirement. But many of us neglect our screening tests. Does the saying 'I recently had my annual physical examination which I get once every seven years' holds true for you too!

1. **Pap Smear and Pelvic Exam:** Check for cervical cancer. A physician performed pap smear should be administered each year to screen for cervical cancer and other cervical abnormalities. Pap smear should be done once annually after the woman has become sexually active.

2. **Pap Smear Plus HPV DNA Test and Pelvic Exam:** Alternatively, some experts recommend it is a more precise means to check for cervical cancer starting at the age of 30 years, every 3 years.

3. **Breast Self-exam:** Thorough breast self-exams should be practiced monthly to check for any breast or nipple changes that may indicate breast conditions or cancer. They should be done once every month starting at the age of 20 years.

4. **Clinical Breast Exam:** A physician-performed clinic breast exam should be administered every year to help detect breast cancer.

5. **Mammogram:** A mammogram, X-ray exam of the breast, should be performed each year beginning at the age of 40 years to help detect breast cancer in its earliest stages. If you are at a higher risk for the disease, it can be done earlier also as per your physician's advice.

6. **Bone Mineral Density Test:** At 65 years or around the age of menopause; earlier for women with previous fragility fractures, family history of osteoporosis, on medications that cause bone loss or have problems with calcium absorption. Used as an indicator of bone strength and osteoporosis risk.

7. **Skin Exam:** A thorough skin exam should be performed by a physician every year to help detect changes that may indicate skin cancer or other skin conditions.

8. **Fecal Occult Blood Test:** A faecal occult blood test should be performed each year beginning at the age of 50 years to help screen for colon cancer.

9. **Blood Pressure Test:** Blood pressure should be checked by a healthcare provider at least every year. More often if it is high.

10. **Eye Exam:** A thorough eye exam should be performed at least every 1-2 years until the age of 60 years and then every year after that to check for diseases such as

glaucoma. Glaucoma test measures eye pressure and eye health.

11. **Diabetes Test:** A fasting plasma glucose diabetes test should be performed every 3 years to detect diabetes.

12. **Cholesterol Test:** A cholesterol blood test should be performed at least every 5 years. High LDL ('bad') cholesterol, high total cholesterol levels or low HDL ('good') cholesterol levels increase the risk of heart disease and stroke.

13. **Thyroid Hormone Test:** This should be done starting at the age of 35 years every 5 years.

14. **Sigmoidoscopy:** A sigmoidoscopy, examination of the rectum and lower portion of the colon should be performed every 5 years to help screen for colon cancer beginning at the age of 50 years. However, a double contrast barium enema every 5 years or a colonoscopy every 10 years (both beginning at the age of 50 years) may be substituted for the sigmoidoscopy.

15. **Double Contrast Barium Enema:** A double contrast barium enema should be performed every 5 years to help screen for colon cancer beginning at the age of 50. However, a sigmoidoscopy every 5 years or a colonoscopy every 10 years (both beginning at the age of 50) may be substituted for the barium enema.

16. **Colonoscopy:** A colonoscopy, examination of the colon with a flexible, lighted tube called a colonoscope, should be performed every 10 years to help screen for colon cancer beginning at the age of 50 years. However, a sigmoidoscopy every 5 years or a double contrast barium enema every 5 years may be substituted for the colonoscopy. Colonoscopy is an outpatient procedure in which a doctor inserts a long,

flexible instrument, about 1/2 an inch in diameter into the rectum to view the rectum and the entire colon. Many experts say colonoscopy is the most accurate colon cancer screening. However, it can be done more often if there is a history of colon polyps.

17. **FSH Test:** An FSH (follicles stimulating hormone) test may be performed to determine whether a woman is close to or has reached menopause.

18. **Vaccines:**

    i. **Tetanus Booster:** Restores protection against tetanus infection, may be given every 10 years.

    ii. **Pneumonia Vaccine:** Provides lifelong protection against pneumonia; may be given to those with risk factors, such as heart failure, lung disease, alcoholism and others.

    iii. **Influenza Vaccine:** Provides protection against common influenza strains; the vaccine can be given at the age of 50 years or earlier and then repeated annually.

Just because you are not sick does not mean you are healthy, take charge of your health before an illness takes charge of you.

References

Introduction

1. Theories of Ageing, Tutor vista.com, 2008.
2. Welcome to Middle Age: The 12 Steps of Middle Adulthood, Keith Drury, 3 February, 2009, http://www.tuesdaycolumn.com/

Chapter 1 Anatomical and Physiological Changes

1. Aging Changes in Hair and Nails, Review Date: 7 November, 2006. Reviewed by: Sandra W. Cohen, M.D. Private Practice specializing in Geriatrics, Brooklyn, NY, Review provided by VeriMed Healthcare Network.
2. Link to - What Causes Gray Hair?', http://www.disabled-world.com/health/dermatology/hair/gray-hair-causes.php, Reviewed on: 8 October, 2008.
3. Aging Changes in Skin – Overview, David C. Dugdale, III, MD, Professor of Medicine, Division of General Medicine, Department of Medicine, University of Washington, School of Medicine. Reviewed by David Zieve, MD, MHA, Medical Director, A.D.A.M., Inc.
4. Brincat M., E. Versi, C.F. Moniz, Magos A., J. de Trafford and J.W., Studd, Skin Collagen Changes in Postmenopausal Women Receiving different Regimens of Estrogen Therapy, Obstet Gynecol, 1987;70(1):123-7.
5. Skin Care—How Skin Changes With Age? Submitted by – C.D. Mohatta, 2 June, 2006, www. Articletrader.com
6. Women's Health Update by Tori Hudson, ND, Professor, National College of Naturopathic Medicine and Bastyr University, Medical Director, A Woman's Time Author, Women's Encyclopedia of Natural Medicine, 2067 N.W. Lovejoy, Portland, Oregon 97209 USA, 503-222-2322.
7. Our Mouth and Teeth Age, Too, Aetna Dental Plans, Updated 12 January, 2009.
8. Vision Changes after 40 Years of Age How Your Vision Changes as You Age, Gary Heiting, OD, Updated February, 2010.

9. Prakash Thulasimani, Read more at Suite101: Vision Changes after 40 Years of Age: Various Eye Problems Connected with Aging, www.suite 101com, 23 December, 2009.
10. Aging Changes in the Senses, Minaker, K.L., Common Clinical Sequelae of Aging. In: Goldman L, Ausiello D, eds. Cecil Medicine. 23rd ed. Philadelphia, Pa: Saunders; 2007: Chapter 23. Updated on 19 February, 2009, Updated by: David C. Dugdale, III, MD, Professor of Medicine, Division of General Medicine, Department of Medicine, University of Washington, School of Medicine. Also reviewed by David Zieve, MD, MHA, Medical Director, A.D.A.M., Inc
11. A Good Night's Sleep, National Institute on Aging, 25 June, 2007, (April 27, 2009) http://www.niapublications.org/agepages/sleep.asp
12. Bakalar, Nicholas, 'Study Links Falls to Lack of Sleep', New York Times, 16 September, 2008. (April 27, 2009) http://www.nytimes.com/2008/09/16/health/research/16agin.html?scp=7&sq=sleep,%20aging&st=cse
13. 'Changes in Sleep with Age', Harvard Healthy Sleep, 18 December , 2007 (April 27, 2009) http://healthysleep.med.harvard.edu/healthy/science/variations/changes-in-sleep-with-age
14. Elias, Marilyn, 'Age and sleep play catch-up', USA Today, 28 July, 2005. (April 27, 2009) http://www.usatoday.com/news/health/2005-07-27-age-and-insomnia x.htm
15. Kolata, Gina, 'Elderly Become Addicts to Drug-Induced Sleep', New York Times, 2 February, 1992 (April 27, 2009). http://www.nytimes.com/1992/02/02/weekinreview/ideas-trends-elderly-become-addicts-to-drug-induced-sleep.html?scp=21&sq=sleep,%20aging&st=cse
16. —————, 'The Elderly Always Sleep Worse, and Other Myths of Aging,' New York Times, 23 October, 2007. (April 27, 2009) http://www.nytimes.com/2007/10/23/health/23age.html?scp=1&sq=sleep,%20aging&st=cse
17. Kryger, Meir, Andrew Monjan, Donald Bliwise and Sonia Ancoli-Israel, 'Sleep, health and aging: Bridging the gap between science and clinical practice,' Geriatrics, January 2004.
18. Lloyd, Robin, 'Elderly Don't Need as Much Sleep, Study Finds,' Live Science, 24 July, 2008 (April 27, 2009) http://www.livescience.com/health/080724-older-sleep.html
19. —————, 'Lack of Sleep Causes Old Men's Testosterone to Drop,' Live Science, 2 April, 2007 (April 27, 2009) http://www.livescience.com/health/070402 sleep testosterone.html
20. 'Sleep and Aging,' NIH Senior Health, 10 April, 2009 (April 27, 2009) http://nihseniorhealth.gov/sleepandaging/toc.html
21. Yoon, In-Young, F. Kripke, Daniel, A. Elliott Jeffrey, D. Youngstedt, Shawn, M. Rex, Katharine, and L. Hauger, Richard, 'Age-Related Changes of Circadian Rhythms and Sleep-Wake Cycles,' *Journal of the American Geriatrics Society*, August 2003.
22. Shneerson, J.M., M.M., Ohayon, M.A., Carskadon, Sleep and Age, National Institutes of Health, Sleep and Aging, About Sleep, The Mayo Clinic, Senior Health Insomnia, Sleep and Aging, by Mark Stibich, Ph.D., About.com Guide, Updated 30 October, 2008, www.health am network.

23. Aging Changes in the Bones - Muscles-Joints, Reviewed: 11 March, 2002 Reviewed by: Steven Angelo, M.D., Assistant Professor of Medicine, Yale School of Medicine, New Haven, CT. Review provided by VeriMed Healthcare Network. Last reviewed and updated: September 2009, American Academy of Orthopedic Surgeons.
24. Aging Changes in Bones. Updated: 10 August 2008, Updated by: David C. Dugdale, III, MD, Professor of Medicine, Division of General Medicine, Department of Medicine, University of Washington, School of Medicine. Reviewed by David Zieve, MD, MHA, Medical Director, A.D.A.M., Inc.
25. Aging Changes in the Bones - Muscles – Joints, How Stuff Works. Updated: 10 August 2008, Updated by: David C. Dugdale, III, MD, Professor of Medicine, Division of General Medicine, Department of Medicine, University of Washington, School of Medicine. Reviewed by David Zieve, MD, MHA, Medical Director, A.D.A.M., Inc.
26. Aging Changes in the Heart and Blood Vessels, Medlineplus, Schwartz, J.B., Zipes, D.P. Cardiovascular Disease in the Elderly. In: Libby P., Bonow R.O., Mann D.L., Zipes DP, eds. *Braunwald's Heart Disease: A Textbook of Cardiovascular Medicine.* 8th ed. Philadelphia, Pa; Saunders Elsevier; 2007: Chapter 75. Updated: 10 August 2008, Updated by: David C. Dugdale, III, MD, Professor of Medicine, Division of General Medicine, Department of Medicine, University of Washington, School of Medicine. Also reviewed by David Zieve, MD, MHA, Medical Director, A.D.A.M., Inc.
27. Aging and the Brain: How Ageing Changes the brain. www.aarp.org
28. Aging Changes in the Female Reproductive System, Reviewed: 1 August, 2008, Reviewed by: Linda Vorvick, MD, Seattle Site Coordinator, Maternal and Child Health Lecturer, Pathophysiology, MEDEX Northwest Division of Physician Assistant Studies, University of Washington, School of Medicine; Susan Storck, MD, FACOG, Clinical Teaching Faculty, Department of Obstetrics and Gynecology, University of Washington School of Medicine; Chief, Eastside Department of Obstetrics and Gynecology, Group Health Cooperative of Puget Sound, Redmond, WA. Reviewed by David Zieve, MD, MHA, Medical Director, A.D.A.M., Inc.
29. Lane Jay Mercer, M.D. Copyright ©1999, Northwestern University, All Rights Reserved, Edited by the Buehler Center on Aging, McGaw Medical Center, j-webster@northwestern.edu. Updated: 9 June, 1999
30. Lobo RA. Menopause: Endocrinology, Consequences of Estrogen Deficiency, Effects of Hormone Replacement Therapy, Treatment Regimens. In: Katz VL, Lentz GM, Lobo RA, Gershenson DM, eds. *Comprehensive Gynecology.* 5th ed. Philadelphia, Pa: Mosby Elsevier; 2007:

Chapter 3 Cervical Cancer

1. Ferlay, J., Bray, F., Pisani, P., DM: GLOBOCAN 2002: Cancer Incidence, Mortality and Prevalence Worldwide. In IARC Cancer Base No. 5, version 2.0. IARC Press, Lyon; 2004.
2. Sankaranaryanan, R., Buduk, A.M., Rajkumar, R.: Effective Screening Programes for Cervical Cancer in low- and middle-income developing countries. Bull World Health Organ 2001., 79(10):

3. International Agency for Research on Cancer (IARC): Handbooks of Cancer Prevention: Cervix Cancer Screening. Volume 10. Lyon, France: IARC; 2005.
4. American Cancer Society Guidelines for cervical cancer from the website Revised: 26 March, 2008
5. Manuals for training in Cancer Control, National Cancer Control Program, Directorate General of Health Services, Ministry of Health and Family welfare, GOI, Nov, 2005.

Chapter 4 Breast Cancer

1. Bailey and Love's Short Practice of Surgery, 23rd edition, Arnold International Students Edition, London: 2001.
2. Detailed Guide: Breast Cancer What Are the Risk Factors for Breast Cancer? Cancer Reference Information, American Cancer Society, 18 September, 2006.
3. Eliassen, Dr. A. Heather, Postmenopausal Weight Gain Increases Breast Cancer Risk JAMA 2006;296: 193-201.
4. Anderson, G.L., Judd, H.L., Kaunitz, A.M., Barad, D.H., et al., Effects of Estrogen plus Progestin on Gynecologic Cancers and Associated Diagnostic Procedures: The Women's Health Initiative randomized trial. JAMA.2003; 290(13):1739-174
5. Polly, A. Marchbanks, Jill A. McDonald, Hoyt G. Wilson, et. al Oral Contraceptives and the Risk of Breast Cancer, *The New England Journal of Medicine*, Volume 346:2025-2032, June 27, 2002, Number 26
6. Chlebowski, Rowan T., Zhao Chen, Garnet L. Anderson, et. al., Ethinicity and Breast Cancer: Factors Influencing Differences and Outcome, J. National Cancer Institute, Volume 97. No.6, 2005.

Chapter 5 Ovarian Cancer

1. Detailed guide: Ovarian Cancer, American Cancer Society. http://documents.cancer.org/114.00/114.00.pdf. Accessed 20 August, 2008.
2. Goff B. Early Detection of Ovarian Cancer: Role of Symptom Recognition. http://www.uptodate.com/home/index.html, Accessed 19 August, 2008.
3. Carlson, K. J, et. al., Patient Information: Ovarian Cancer Screening. http://www.uptodate.com/home/index.html, Accessed 19 August, 2008.
4. Ovarian Cancer: Treatment Guidelines for Patients, National Comprehensive Cancer Network and the American Cancer Society, http://www.cancer.org/downloads/CRI/NCCN Ovarian Cancer 2007, Accessed 19 August, 2008.
5. Herzog, T.J., et. al., Patient information: Ovarian Cancer Treatment. http://www.uptodate.com/home/index.html, Accessed 19 August , 2008.
6. Timothy Moynihan (expert review), Mayo Clinic, Rochester, Minn., 28 August, 2008.
7. Ovarian Cancer Symptoms, Early Warning Signs, and Risk Factors www.medicinenet.com, Reviewed: 14 June, 2007, Medical Author: Melissa Conrad

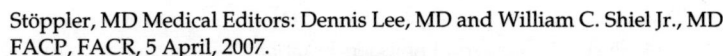

Stöppler, MD Medical Editors: Dennis Lee, MD and William C. Shiel Jr., MD, FACP, FACR, 5 April, 2007.
8. Ovarian Cancer from www.imaginis.com, Updated: 10 January, 2008
9. National Toxicology Program, "Toxicology and Carcinogenesis Studies of Talc (GAS No. 14807-96-6) in F344/N Rats and B6C3F, Mice (Inhalation studies)." *Technical Report Series* No. 421, September 1993.
10 Harlow, B.L., D.W. Cramer, D.A. Bell, W.R. Welch, "Perineal Exposure to Talc and Ovarian Cancer Risk", *Obstetrics & Gynecology*, 80: 19-26, 1992.
11. Ovarian Cancer, www.mayoclinic.com, 11 November, 2008

Chapter 6 Cancer of the Uterus

1. National Cancer Institute, What You Need to Know about Cancer of the Uterus, www. Cancer.gov, posted 30 July, 2001, updated 16 September, 2002.
2. Brachytherapy, 19 March, 2008, PMID: 18358790
3. American Cancer Society, Uterine Sarcomas — Hormonal Therapy, Accessed 25 May, 2007.
4. Santin, A.D., S. Bellone, J.J. Roman, J.K. McKenney,   S. Pecorelli, 2008. 'Trastuzumab treatment in patients with advanced or recurrent endometrial carcinoma overexpressing HER2/neu, Int. J. Gynaecol Obstet 102 (2): 128–31. doi:10.1016/j.ijgo.2008.04.008, PMID 18555254.
5. National Cancer Guidance Steering Group, Improving Outcomes in Gynaecological Cancers: The Research Evidence London: NHS Executive, Department of Health, 1999
6. American Cancer Society, Endometrial Cancer Resource Center.

Chapter 7 Fibroids

1. DE Larson, Mayo Family Health Book, 1996.
2. Uerine fibroids, www.mayoclinic.com, 15 June, 2007
3. Goto, A., S. Takeuchi, K. Sugimura, and T. Maruo 2002, 'Usefulness of Gd-DTPA contrast-enhanced dynamic MRI and serum determination of LDH and its isozymes in the differential diagnosis of leiomyosarcoma from degenerated leiomyoma of the uterus', Int. J. Gynecol. Cancer, 12 (4): 354–61. doi:10.1046/j.1525-1438.2002.01086.x. PMID 12144683.
4. Indman, Paul D., 'Hysteroscopic Myomectomy for Removal of Uterine Fibroids', personal web page, 2001
5. Polena, V., et. al., 'Long-term Results of Hysteroscopic Myomectomy in 235 patients', European Journal of Obstetrics & Gynecology and Reproductive Biology, 130 (2007): 232-237.
6 Agdi, M., and T. Tulandi, 'Endoscopic Management of Uterine Fibroids', Best Practice & Research Clinical Obstetrics & Gynecology, online publication, 4 March, 2008.
7. American Society of Reproductive Medicine Patient Booklet: Uterine Fibroids, 2003.

8. Howkins & Bourne, Shaw's Textbook of Gynaecology, 14th edition.
9. V.G, Shirish N. Daftary, Publisher: Else Shaw's Textbook of Gynaecology, Padubidri.

Chapter 8   Uterine Prolapse

1. Lawrence Impeypg Blackwell publishing, *Prolapse of Uterus and Vagina, Obstetrics and Gynaecology*, 2nd edition.
2. WEB HEALTH MD, 19 April, 2009
3. MEDLINEPLUS Updated: 6 June, 2006, References for uterine prolapse.
4. Medline Uterine Prolapse, Author: Thomas Mailhot, MD, Staff Physician, Department of Emergency Medicine, University of Southern California, Los Angeles County Coauthor(s): Allison J Richard, MD, Instructor of Clinical Emergency Medicine, Keck School of Medicine, University of Southern California; Consulting Staff, Department of Emergency Medicine, LAC-USC Medical Center Updated: May 24, 2006.

Chapter 9   Dysfunctional Uterine Bleeding

1. Bayer, S.R., A.H. DeCherney, *Clinical Manifestations and Treatment of Dysfunctional Uterine Bleeding*, JAMA 1993, 269:1823-8.
2. Fayez, J.A., *Dysfunctional Uterine Bleeding*, Am Fam Physician, 1982, 25:109-15.
3. Johnson, C.A., Making Sense of Dysfunctional Uterine Bleeding, Am Fam Physician, 1991, 44:149-57
4. Howkins & Bourne, Shaw's Textbook of Gynaecology, 14th edition.
5. Padubidri V.G., Shirish N., Daftary Publisher: Else, Shaw's Textbook of Gynaecology.

Chapter 10   Menopause

1. Minkin, et. al., 1997, *What Every Woman Needs to Know about Menopause*, Yale University Press, ISBN 0300072619
2. Twiss, J.J., J. Wegner, M. Hunter, M., Kelsay, M., Rathe-Hart, W., Salado, 2007, "Perimenopausal Symptoms, Quality of Life and Health behaviors in users and nonusers of hormone therapy". J Am Acad Nurse Pract 19 (11): 602–13. doi:10.1111/j.1745-7599.2007.00260.x. PMID 17970860. http://www.blackwell-synergy.com/openurl?genre=article&sid=nlm:pubmed&issn=1041-2972&date=2007&volume=19&issue=11&spage=602.
3. Sengupta, A., *The Emergence of Menopause in India*, Climateric, 2003, June; 6(2);92-5
4. Pien, G.W, M.D. Sammel, E.W. Freeman, Lin H., DeBlasis T.L. July 2008, "Predictors of sleep quality in women in the menopausal transition". Sleep 31 (7): 991–9. PMID 18652094

5. Seifer, David B., Elizabeth A. Kennard, (Menopause Endocrinology and Management) Menopause: Endocrinology and Management, Edition: illustrated, Humana Press, 1999.
6. The National Institute of Aging provides information on menopause at http://www.nih.gov/nia/http://www.imaginis.com/womenshealth/menopause.asp
7. May 31, 2001 American College of Obstetricians and Gynecologists (ACOG) news release, "It's 'Buyer Beware' with Alternative Botanical Treatments for Menopausal Symptoms, Says ACOG," http://www.acog.org. Contact the ACOG for more information on the new guidelines entitled "Use of Botanicals for Management of Menopausal Symptoms.
8. Syamala, T.S. and M. Sivakami of ISEC used data from the National Family Health Survey, conducted in 1988 and 1999,
9. (India together) Neeta lal, 8 March, 2007.
10. Menopause .www.medicinenet.com Medical Author: Melissa Conrad Stöppler, MD Medical Editor: William C. Shiel Jr., MD, FACP, FACR

Chapter 11 Hormone Replacement Therapy (HRT)

1. UAB Health system
2. Rossouw , J.E, G.L., Anderson , R.L., Prentice, et. al. (2002). "Risks and benefits of estrogen plus progestin in healthy postmenopausal women: principal results From the Women's Health Initiative randomized controlled trial". JAMA 288 (3): 321–33. doi:10.1001/jama.288.3.321. PMID 12117397.
3. Anderson, G.L., M. Limacher, M., A.R. Assaf, et al. (2004). "Effects of Conjugated Equine Estrogen in Postmenopausal Women with Hysterectomy: The Women's Health Initiative Randomized Controlled Trial". JAMA 291 (14): 1701–12. doi:10.1001/jama.291.14.1701. PMID 15082697.
4. Manson, J.E., P.H.J. Hsia, K.C. Johnson, J.E. Rossouw, A.R. Assaf, N. L. Lasser, N.L. Trevisan, M., Black, H.R., Heckbert, S.R., Detrano, R., Strickland, O.L., Wong, N.D., Crouse, J.R., Stein, E. & Cushman, M. (2003). "Estrogen plus Progestin and the Risk of Coronary Heart Disease". The New England Journal of Medicine 349 (6): 523–534. doi:10.1056/NEJMoa030808. PMID 12904517.
5. Scarabin PY, Oger E, Plu-Bureau G (2003). "Differential association of oral and transdermal oestrogen-replacement therapy with venous thromboembolism risk". Lancet 362 (9382): 428–32. doi:10.1016/S0140-6736(03)14066-4. PMID 12927428.
6. Anderson, G.L, M. Limacher, A.R. Assaf, et. al. (2004). "Effects of conjugated equine estrogen in postmenopausal women with hysterectomy: the Women's Health Initiative randomized controlled trial". JAMA 291 (14): 1701–12. doi:10.1001/jama.291.14.1701. PMID 15082697.
7. Stefanick, M.L., G.L. Anderson, K.L. Margolis, et. al. (2006). "Effects of conjugated equine estrogens on breast cancer and mammography screening in postmenopausal women with hysterectomy". JAMA 295 (14): 1647–57. doi:10.1001/jama.295.14.1647. PMID 16609086.

8. Hulley SB, Grady D (2004). "The WHI estrogen-alone trial—do things look any better?". JAMA 291 (14): 1769–71. doi:10.1001/jama.291.14.1769. PMID 15082705.
9. B. Stephen, G. Timothy, Hormone Replacement Therapy, retrieved January 15, 2007, http://www.quackwatch.org/03HealthPromotion/hrt.html, Hormone Replacement Therapy FAQ's, retrieved January 15, 2007, http://womenshealth.about.com/library/blhrt.htm
10. Hormone Replacement Therapy, Medical Encyclopedia, retrieved January 15, 2007, http://www.nlm.nih.gov/medlineplus/ency/article/007111.htm
11. HRT in the news, retrieved January 15, 2007, http://www.cwhn.ca/resources/menopause/hrt-glance.html
12. Writing Group for the Women's Health Initiative Investigators. Risks and benefits of estrogen plus progestin in healthy postmenopausal women: principal results from the Women's Health Initiative randomized controlled trial. JAMA 2002; 288: 321-33.
13. Brown, Ann J., M.D. Hormone Replacement Therapy & Menopause, Duke University Medical Centre. February 2009
14. Hormone Therapy and Menopause by Elizabeth Santoro, RN, MPH, Maushami DeSoto, PhD, and Jae Hong Lee, MD, MPH
15. Clarke CA, Glaser SL, Uratsu CS, Selby JV, Kushi LH, Herrinton LJ (November 2006). "Recent declines in hormone therapy utilization and breast cancer incidence: clinical and population-based evidence". J. Clin. Oncol. 24 (33): e49–50. doi:10.1200/JCO.2006.08.6504. PMID 17114650.
16. Ravdin PM, Cronin KA, Howlader N, et al. (April 2007). "The decrease in breast-cancer incidence in 2003 in the United States". N. Engl. J. Med. 356 (16): 1670–4. doi:10.1056/NEJMsr070105. PMID 17442911.
17. Glass AG, Lacey JV, Carreon JD, Hoover RN (August 2007). "Breast cancer incidence, 1980-2006: combined roles of menopausal hormone therapy, screening mammography, and estrogen receptor status". J. Natl. Cancer Inst. 99 (15): 1152–61. doi:10.1093/jnci/djm059. PMID 17652280

Chapter 12 Urinary Incontinence

1. www.Mayoclinic,12th June 2008Kegel'sexercise. How to strengthen pelvic floor muscles.
2. UAB Health system
3. Textbook Of Female Urology And Urogynecology, Second Edition .- Oct 2005) by Linda Cardozo, David R. Staskin, Cardozo CardozoPublisher: Informa Healthcare .
4. Norton P, et al. Urinary incontinence in women. The Lancet. 2006;367(9504):57-67.
5. National Kidney and Urologic Diseases Information Clearinghouse: Incontinence (Loss of Bladder Control) http://kidney.niddk.nih.gov/kudiseases/topics/incontinence.asp
6. National Association For Continence http://www.nafc.org/
7. American Urogynecologic Society http://www.mypelvichealth.org

Chapter 13 Hypertension (High Blood Pressure)

1. Written by familydoctor.org editorial staff. American Academy of Family Physicians Reviewed/Updated: 11/06 Created: 09/00
2. Checking Your Blood Pressure at Home Clinical Diabetes 22:32, 2004© American Diabetes Association ®, Inc., 2004
3. Hypertension. www.mayoclinic.com
4. Tips to Monitor Your Blood Pressure at Home, Simeon Margolis, M.D., Ph.D.- Posted on Fri, Sep 22, 2006, 12:30 pm www.johnhopkins medicine.org
5. Heart and stroke foundation of Canada. How to measure your blood pressure at home, Reviewed, Dec 2008.
6. Davidson's Principles & Practice Of Medicine Jul 2006), 20th edition Nicholas A. Boon, Nicki R. Colledge, Brian R. Walker Publisher: Churchill Livingstone Harrison's Principles of Internal Medicine textbook by McGraw-Hill Companies; Stone, Richard M.; Fauci, Anthony S.; (Author) 17th edition

Chapter 14 Diabetes

1. www.Mayoclinic.com, Diabetes Mellitus, 9th April, 2009.
2. Zimmet P, Alberti KG, Shaw J (December 2001). "Global and societal implications of the diabetes epidemic". Nature 414 (6865): 782–7. doi:10.1038/414782a. PMID 11742409. http://www.nature.com/nature/journal/v414/n6865/abs/414782a.html. Retrieved on 2008-07-19.
3. World Health Organization. "Definition, diagnosis and classification of diabetes mellitus and its complications: Report of a WHO Consultation. Part 1. Diagnosis and classification of diabetes mellitus". http://www.who.int/diabetes/publications/en/. Retrieved on 2007-05-29.
4. Your guide to diabetes: Type 1 and type 2. National Institute of Diabetes and Digestive and Kidney Diseases. http://diabetes.niddk.nih.gov/dm/pubs/type1and2/index.htm. Accessed April 1, 2009.
5. Diabetes Mellitus (DM). The Merck Manuals: The Merck Manual for Healthcare Professionals. http://www.merck.com/mmpe/sec12/ch158/ch158b.html#sec12-ch158-ch158b-1105. Accessed April 2, 2009.

Chapter 15 Raised Cholesterol Level (Hypercholesterolemia)

1. Brunzell JD, Davidson M, Furberg CD, Goldberg RB, Howard BV, Stein JH, Witztum JL (April 2008). "Lipoprotein management in patients with cardiometabolic risk: consensus statement from the American Diabetes Association and the American College of Cardiology Foundation". Diabetes Care 31 (4): 811–22. doi:10.2337/dc08-9018. PMID 18375431.
2. Durrington P (August 2003). "Dyslipidaemia". Lancet 362 (9385): 717–31. doi:10.1016/S0140-6736(03)14234-1. PMID 12957096.
3. Report of the National Cholesterol Education Program Expert Panel on Detection, Evaluation, and Treatment of High Blood Cholesterol in

Adults. The Expert Panel". Arch. Intern. Med. 148 (1): 36–69. January 1988. doi:10.1001/archinte.148.1.36. PMID 3422148

4.. "High blood cholesterol: what you need to know". National cholesterol education program. http://www.nhlbi.nih.gov/health/public/heart/chol/wyntk.htm. Retrieved on 2008-10-24.

5. "How To Get Your Cholesterol Tested". American Heart Association. http://www.americanheart.org/presenter.jhtml?identifier=541. Retrieved on 2009

6. High blood cholesterol. National Heart Lung and Blood Institute. http://www.nhlbi.nih.gov/health/dci/Diseases/Hbc/HBC_all.html. Accessed Jan. 5, 2009.

7. Women and cholesterol. American Heart Association. http://www.americanheart.org/presenter.jhtml?identifier=185. Accessed Jan. 5, 2009.

Chapter 16 Obesity

1. Middle Aged Women Hate Their Bodies And Are Developing Eating DisordersWritten by: Christian Nordqvist Editor: Medical News Today
2. Haslam DW, James WP (2005). "Obesity". Lancet 366 (9492): 1197–209. doi:10.1016/S0140-6736(05)67483-1. PMID 16198769.
3. NICE 2006 p.10–11
4. Barness LA, Opitz JM, Gilbert-Barness E (December 2007). "Obesity: genetic, molecular, and environmental aspects". Am. J. Med. Genet. A 143A (24): 3016–34. doi:10.1002/ajmg.a.32035. PMID 18000969.
5. Woodhouse R (2008). "Obesity in art: A brief overview". Front Horm Res 36: 271–86. doi:10.1159/000115370. PMID 18230908. http://books.google.ca/books?id=nXRU4Ea1aMkC&pg=PA271&lpg=PA271&dq=Obesity+in+art:+a+brief+overview&source=web&ots=G2ofZTj_r&sig=7HbW8aAnoQ-RIwt09ocD3xOHJZU&hl=en&sa=X&oi=book_result&resnum=5&ct=result#PPA271,M1.
6. Sweeting HN (2007). "Measurement and definitions of obesity in childhood and adolescence: A field guide for the uninitiated". Nutr J 6: 32. doi:10.1186/1475-2891-6-32. PMID 17963490. http://www.nutritionj.com/content/6/1/32. NHLBI p.xiv
7. Schwarz, Steven (November 1, 2007). "Obesity". emedicine. http://www.emedicine.com/med/TOPIC1653.HTM. Retrieved on 2008-09-30.
8. U.S. Preventive Services Task Force Evidence Syntheses (2000). HSTAT: Guide to Clinical Preventive Services, 3rd Edition: Recommendations and Systematic Evidence Reviews, Guide to Community Preventive Services. http://www.ncbi.nlm.nih.gov/books/bv.fcgi?rid=hstat3.section.36199.
9. Jebb and Wells 2005 p.20
10. Mei Z, Grummer-Strawn LM, Pietrobelli A, Goulding A, Goran MI, Dietz WH (01 Jun 2002). "Validity of body mass index compared with other body-composition screening indexes for the assessment of body fatness in children and adolescents". Am J Clin Nutr 75 (6): 978–85. PMID 12036802. http://www.ajcn.org/cgi/content/full/75/6/978.

References

11. Gabriel I Uwaifo (June 19, 2006). "Obesity". emedicine.com. http://www.emedicine.com/med/TOPIC1653.HTM. Retrieved on 2008-09-29.
12. Kanazawa M, Yoshiike N, Osaka T, Numba Y, Zimmet P, Inoue S (December 2002). "Criteria and classification of obesity in Japan and Asia-Oceania". Asia Pac J Clin Nutr 11 Suppl 8: S732–S737. doi:10.1046/j.1440-6047.11.s8.19.x. PMID 12534701. http://www3.interscience.wiley.com/resolve/openurl?genre=article&sid=nlm:pubmed&issn=0964-7058&date=2002&volume=11&issue=&spage=S732.
13. Bei-Fan Z (December 2002). "Predictive values of body mass index and waist circumference for risk factors of certain related diseases in Chinese adults: study on optimal cut-off points of body mass index and waist circumference in Chinese adults". Asia Pac J Clin Nutr 11 Suppl 8: S685–93. doi:10.1046/j.1440-6047.11.s8.9.x. PMID 12534691. http://www3.interscience.wiley.com/resolve/openurl?genre=article&sid=nlm:pubmed&issn=0964-7058&date=2002&volume=11&issue=&spage=S685.
14. Yusuf S, Hawken S, Ounpuu S, Dans T, Avezum A, Lanas F, McQueen M, Budaj A, Pais P, Varigos J, Lisheng L, INTERHEART Study Investigators. (2004). "Effect of potentially modifiable risk factors associated with myocardial infarction in 52 countries (the INTERHEART study): Case-control study". Lancet 364: 937–52. doi:10.1016/S0140-6736(04)17018-9. PMID 15364185.
15. Strychar I (January 2006). "Diet in the management of weight loss". CMAJ 174 (1): 56–63. doi:10.1503/cmaj.045037. PMID 16389240. PMC: 1319349. http://www.cmaj.ca/cgi/content/full/174/1/56.
16. Wing, Rena R; Phelan, Suzanne (01 July 2005). "Science-Based Solutions to Obesity: What are the Roles of Academia, Government, Industry, and Health Care? Proceedings of a symposium, Boston, Massachusetts, USA, 10–11 March 2004 and Anaheim, California, USA, 2 October 2004". Am. J. Clin. Nutr. 82 (1 Suppl): 207S–273S. PMID 16002825. http://www.ajcn.org/cgi/content/full/82/1/222S.
17. Weiss EC, Galuska DA, Kettel Khan L, Gillespie C, Serdula MK (July 2007). "Weight regain in U.S. adults who experienced substantial weight loss, 1999–2002". Am J Prev Med 33 (1): 34–40. doi:10.1016/j.amepre.2007.02.040. PMID 17572309.
18. Anderson JW, Konz EC, Frederich RC, Wood CL (01 November 2001). "Long-term weight-loss maintenance: A meta-analysis of US studies". Am. J. Clin. Nutr. 74 (5): 579–84. PMID 11684524. http://www.ajcn.org/cgi/content/full/74/5/579.
19. Williamson DF, Pamuk E, Thun M, Flanders D, Byers T, Heath C (June 1995). "Prospective study of intentional weight loss and mortality in never-smoking overweight US white women aged 40–64 years". Am. J. Epidemiol. 141 (12): 1128–41. PMID 7771451.
20. Sacks FM, Bray GA, Carey VJ, et al (February 2009). "Comparison of weight-loss diets with different compositions of fat, protein, and carbohydrates". N. Engl. J. Med. 360 (9): 859–73. doi:10.1056/NEJMoa0804748. PMID 19246357.
21. Bravata DM, Sanders L, Huang J, et al. (April 2003). "Efficacy and safety of low-carbohydrate diets: A systematic review". JAMA 289 (14): 1837–50. doi:10.1001/jama.289.14.1837. PMID 12684364.

22. Hession M, Rolland C, Kulkarni U, Wise A, Broom J (January 2009). "Systematic review of randomized controlled trials of low-carbohydrate vs. low-fat/low-calorie diets in the management of obesity and its comorbidities". Obes Rev 10 (1): 36–50. doi:10.1111/j.1467-789X.2008.00518.x. PMID 18700873.
23. Gwinup G (1987). "Weight loss without dietary restriction: Efficacy of different forms of aerobic exercise". Am J Sports Med 15 (3): 275–9. doi:10.1177/036354658701500317. PMID 3618879.
24. Sahlin K, Sallstedt EK, Bishop D, Tonkonogi M (December 2008). "Turning down lipid oxidation during heavy exercise—what is the mechanism?". J. Physiol. Pharmacol. 59 Suppl 7: 19–30. PMID 19258655. http://www.jpp.krakow.pl/journal/archive/1208_s7/pdf/19_1208_s7_article.pdf.
25. Shaw K, Gennat H, O'Rourke P, Del Mar C (2006). "Exercise for overweight or obesity". Cochrane database of systematic reviews (Online) (4): CD003817. doi:10.1002/14651858.CD003817.pub3. PMID 17054187.
26. Lee L, Kumar S, Leong LC (February 1994). "The impact of five-month basic military training on the body weight and body fat of 197 moderately to severely obese Singaporean males aged 17 to 19 years". Int. J. Obes. Relat. Metab. Disord. 18 (2): 105–9. PMID 8148923.
27. Bessesen DH (June 2008). "Update on obesity". J. Clin. Endocrinol. Metab. 93 (6): 2027–34. doi:10.1210/jc.2008-0520. PMID 18539769.
28. Bravata DM, Smith-Spangler C, Sundaram V, et al (November 2007). "Using pedometers to increase physical activity and improve health: a systematic review". JAMA : the journal of the American Medical Association 298 (19): 2296–304. doi:10.1001/jama.298.19.2296. PMID 18029834.
29. "www.paho.org". Pan American Health Organization. http://www.paho.org/English/DD/PIN/ePersp001_article01.htm. Retrieved on January 10, 2009.
30. "WIN - Publication - Prescription Medications for the Treatment of Obesity". National Institute of Diabetes and Digestive and Kidney Diseases (NIDDK). National Institutes of Health. http://win.niddk.nih.gov/publications/prescription.htm#fdameds. Retrieved on January 14, 2009.
31. Rucker D, Padwal R, Li SK, Curioni C, Lau DC (2007). "Long term pharmacotherapy for obesity and overweight: Updated meta-analysis". BMJ 335 (7631): 1194–99. doi:10.1136/bmj.39385.413113.25. PMID 18006966.
32. Encinosa WE, Bernard DM, Chen CC, Steiner CA (2006). "Healthcare utilization and outcomes after bariatric surgery". Medical care 44 (8): 706–12. doi:10.1097/01.mlr.0000220833.89050.ed. PMID 16862031.
33. Snow V, Barry P, Fitterman N, Qaseem A, Weiss K (2005). "Pharmacologic and surgical management of obesity in primary care: A clinical practice guideline from the American College of Physicians". Ann Intern Med 142 (7): 525–31. PMID 15809464. Fulltext.
34. Baron M (November 2004). "Commercial weight-loss programs". Health Care Food Nutr Focus 21 (11): 8–9. PMID 15559885. http://meta.wkhealth.com/pt/pt-core/template-journal/lwwgateway/media/landingpage.htm?issn=1090-2260&volume=21&issue=11&spage=8.
35. What is the evidence, reasons for and impact of weight gain during menopause? Med J Aust 2000; 173 Suppl 6 November: S100-S101

Chapter 17 Women and Heart Disease

1. WHO REPORT SHAPING THE FUTURE, Geneva,WHO;2003.
2. National Heart, Lung, and Blood Institute of the National Institutes of Health (NIH).uab health systems. Medicine that touches the world. Women and Heart disease.
3. Heart Disease and Heart Attacks: What Women Need to Know Written by familydoctor.org editorial staff. American Academy of Family PhysiciansReviewed/Updated: 11/06 www.familydoctor.org
4. Mosca L, et al. Evidence-based guidelines for cardiovascular disease prevention in women: 2007 update. Circulation. 2007;49:1230.
5. Frequently asked questions: Heart disease. U.S. Department of Health and Human Services, Office on Women's Health. http://www.4woman.gov/faq/heart-disease.pdf. Accessed Dec. 10, 2008.
6. Li TY, et al. Obesity as Compared With Physical Activity in Predicting Risk of Coronary Heart Disease in Women. Circulation. 2006;113:499.

Chapter 18 Osteoporosis

1. Food and Nutrition Board, Institute of Medicine, National Academy of Sciences, 1997
2. An Atlas of OsteoporosisBy Stevenson, John C. (Author), Marsh, Michael S. (Author) The Third editionPublisher: Informa Healthcare
3. National Institutes of Health (NIH): Osteoporosis and Related Bone Diseases, National Resource Center http://www.osteo.org
4. National Osteoporosis Foundation http://www.nof.org/
5. www.mayoclinic.com
6. www.xplain.com
7. www.imaginis.com

Chapter 19 Osteoarthritis

1. Mayo clinic. guide to managing arthritis.

Chapter 20 Urinary Tract Infection (UTI)

1. Perrotta C, Aznar M, Mejia R, Albert X, Ng CW. Oestrogens for preventing recurrent urinary tract infection in postmenopausal women. Cochrane Database Syst Rev. 2008 Apr 16;(2):CD005131.
2. www.university of Maryland.edu
3. Raz R.Postmenopausal women with recurrent UTI.Int J Antimicrob Agents.2001 Apr;17(4):269-71
4. M.Louis Moy,Uro Today Risk factors for UTI in postmenopausal Women, Tuesday.01.February2005

5. American Association of Sexuality Educators, Counselors and Therapists http://www.aasect.org

Chapter 22 Mental and Psychological Problems

1. Fewer Middle-Aged Women Happy, Study Says More Depression Found Among Those For Caring For Elderly Relatives NEW YORK, Nov. 14, 2006 | by Caitlin A. Johnson
2. One in four middle-aged women suffering depression Tuesday, 27 January 2009 ,Telegraph, Belfast BT Woman.
3. Women's Depression Rate Is HigherBy DANIEL GOLEMANPublished: Thursday, December 6, 1990
4. E max health Obesity, Depression Often Coexist In Middle-Aged Women Submitted by hareyan on Jan 16th, 2008
5. Social Anxiety And Stress www.Life positive.com
6. Major depressive disorder. In: Diagnostic and Statistical Manual of Mental Disorders DSM-IV-TR. 4th ed. Arlington, Va.: American Psychiatric Association; 2000. http://www.psychiatryonline.com. Accessed March 9, 2009.

Chapter 24 Sexual Health

1. Sexuality Older women's sexuality. Lesley A Yee and Kendra J Sundquist MJA 2003; 178 (12): 640-643
2. Web MD, Healthy aging health center 11 th may 2009
3. www.mayoclinic.com women's health Women's sexual health: How to reach sexual fulfillment, April 2, 2009.
4. American Association of Sexuality Educators, Counselors and Therapists http://www.aasect.org

Chapter 25 Pregnancy After 40

1. Has anyone out there over 36 gotten pregnant? Women's Health Matters http://www.womenshealthmatters.ca/index.cfm
2. Information about amniocentesis and chorionic villi sampling. University of Pennsylvania Health Systems website. Available at: http://www.obgyn.upenn.edu/genetics/inforforamnandcvs.html.
3. March of Dimes website. Available at: http://www.modimes.org/.
4. Nurses Portal website. Available at: http://www.virtualnurse.com/.
5. Pregnancy rate among women over 40 reaches record highThe Guardian, Friday 29 February 2008 John Carvel and Sarah Boseley.Published: Monday,12-Feb-2007
6. What are Your Chances of Getting Pregnant After 35? Rachel Gurevich, About.com Updated: November 12, 2008

7. Moving Through Life - Women's Health Fitness Programs Facing Your Pregnancy After 40,Posted at December 10th, 2008
8. Information about amniocentesis and chorionic villi sampling. University of Pennsylvania Health Systems website. Available at: http://www.obgyn.upenn.edu/genetics/inforforamnandcvs.html. 8.March of Dimes website. Available at: http://www.modimes.org .
9. Nurses Portal website. Available at: http://www.virtualnurse.com .
10. Watch Out for Pregnancy Pitfalls After Age 40 Baptist Health System by: Roy J. Ducote MD Last reviewed August 2007 by Jeff Andrews, MD, FRCSC, FACOG
11. Women's health: special problems with pregnancy over 40 Issues and problems for pregnant women over 40.Essortment Written by Ann MacDonald 2002

Chapter 26   Contraception After 40

1. Frank O, Bianchi PG, Campana A. The end of fertility: age, fecundity and fecundability in women. J Biosoc Sci 1994; 26:3:349-68.
2. Contraception after 40 Kirsten Braun and reviewed by the Editorial Committee in June 2006. Women's health Queensland wide Inc. Last Modified: June 13, 2006.
3. Yusuf F & Siedlecky S. Contraceptive use in Australia : Evidence from the 1995 National Health Survey Australian and New Zealand Journal of Obstetrics & Gynaecology 1999; 30:1:58-62
4. AMA Queensland. Australian men carry the load for contraception [media release] October 27 2004
5. Szarewski, A & Guillebaud J. Contraception: A User's Handbook Oxford University Press 1998; 36-41
6. Guillebaud, J. Contraception: Your Questions Answered. Edinburgh: Churchill Livingstone 2004
7. Guillebaud, J. Ibid; 431
8. Guillebaud, J. Ibid; 68
9. Contraception and the Mature Woman http://www.patient.co.uk/showdoc/40024661 [website] date accessed: 10 January 2006

Chapter 27   Physical Fitness

1. National Women's Health Report , Dec, 2002   by Pamela Peeke
2. Hitting the Gym After 40 - Redefining the Aging Process by Diane Fields, ISSA Certified Fitness Trainer, Specialist in Performance Nutrition, Fitness writer www.legendaryfitness.com
3. US dept of Health and Human Services, Public Health service, Centers Control and Prevention, National center for chronic diseases, Prevention and Health Promotion, Division of Nutrition and Physical Activity. Promoting Physical activity; a guide for community action, Champaign IL; Human

Kinetics, 1999(Table adapted from Ainsworth BE,Haskell WL,Leon AS, et al. Compendium of physical activities: classification of energy costs of human activities. Medicine and Science in Sports and Exercise 1993;25(1):71-80.
4. National Institute on Aging. Age Page. Exercise: Feeling Fit for Life. 1998.
5. Fitness tips for menopause: Why physical activity matters www. Mayoclinic. com

Chapter 28 Diet

References: "Choose Your Foods: Exchange Lists for Diabetes," which is the basis of a meal planning system, 2008 American Diabetes Association and American Dietetic Association.

1. Reading food labels. American Diabetes Association. http://www.diabetes.org/nutrition-and-recipes/nutrition/foodlabel.jsp. Accessed Aug. 7, 2008.
2. Taking a closer look at the label. American Diabetes Association. http://www.diabetes.org/nutrition-and-recipes/nutrition/foodlabel/closer-look.jsp. Accessed Aug. 7, 2008.
3. Nutrient content claims & Percent (&) Daily Value. American Diabetes Association. http://www.diabetes.org/nutrition-and-recipes/nutrition/foodlabel/nutrient-content-claims.jsp. Accessed Aug. 7, 2008.
4. Extra tips for people with diabetes. American Diabetes Association. http://www.diabetes.org/nutrition-and-recipes/nutrition/foodlabel/extra-tips.jsp. Accessed Aug. 7, 2008.
5. Food and meal planning. U.S. Food and Drug Administration. http://www.fda.gov/Diabetes/food.html#4. Accessed Aug. 8, 2008.
6. Virtual grocery store: Food labels. American Diabetes Association. http://vgs.diabetes.org/planningmeals/foodlabels.jsp. Accessed Aug. 8, 2008.
7. Diet Tips for Middle Aged Women,National Institutes of Health,National Heart, Lung and Blood Institute April 06, 2009 by Teresa Stacey.
8. NHLBI Study Finds DASH Diet and Reduced Sodium Lowers Blood Pressure For All
9. Dr. George Jacob,Heart Infocenter. Hypertension (High blood pressure) Holisticonline.com
10. Your guide to lowering your blood pressure with DASH. DASH eating plan: Lower your blood pressure. U.S. Department of Health and Human Sciences, National Institutes of Health, National Heart, Lung, and Blood Institute, NIH Publication No. 06-4082,originally printed 1998, revised April 2006.

Chapter 29 Cosmetic Surgery

1. Why is Cosmetic Surgery Popular With Older Women? By Alice Williams
2. Williams, Alice "Why is Cosmetic Surgery Popular With Older Women?." Why is Cosmetic Surgery Popular With Older Women?. 27 Aug. 2008. EzineArticles.com. 6 Jun 2009 <http://ezinearticles.com/?Why-is-Cosmetic-Surgery-Popular-With-Older-Women?&id=1446824>.

References

3. Liposuction 101 Consumer guide to plastic surgery.By Denise Mann; reviewed by Peter Fodor, MD, FACS Source: FDA website."What Are the Risks or Complications Associated with Liposuction?"
4. Liposuction, Is it Right For You? By Kalona Karrington
5. Karrington, Kalona "Liposuction, Is it Right For You?." Liposuction, Is it Right For You?. 3 Jun. 2009. EzineArticles.com. 6 Jun 2009 <http://ezinearticles.com/?Liposuction,-Is-it-Right-For-You?&id=2430242>.
6. MLA Style Citation: Aaronson, A "Tummy Tuck - How Long Should You Wait After Childbirth to Get One?." Tummy Tuck - How Long Should You Wait After Childbirth to Get One?. 16 Mar. 2009. EzineArticles.com. 6 Jun 2009 <http://ezinearticles.com/?Tummy-Tuck—How-Long-Should-You-Wait-After-Childbirth-to-Get-One?&id=2105603
7. What You Need to Know About Tummy Tuck
8. Reviewed by Richard J. Greco, MD, FACSTYou're the proud mother of two children and [page updated October 2008] Consumer guide to plastic surgery
9. Facelift Variations Reviewed by Scott R. Miller, MD, FACS Consumer guide to plastic surgery Face lift Variations page updated October 2008]
10. Stretch Marks Reviewed by Mitchel Goldman, MD and Scott R. Miller, MD, FACS Scott R. Miller, MD, FACS, is a member of the editorial advisory board for Consumer Guide to Plastic Surgery. A board-certified plastic surgeon, Dr. Miller practices in La Jolla, California. [More about Dr. Miller.] [page updated June 2008]
11. Female Hair Loss: Causes, Treatment and Prevention By Denise Mann; reviewed by Neil Sadick, MD,March 2009,updated,consumer guide to plastic surgery Harel, Tom "Breast Augmentation - 5 Things Women Should Know." Breast Augmentation - 5 Things Women Should Know. 22 Feb. 2009. EzineArticles.com. 6 Jun 2009 <http://ezinearticles.com/?Breast-Augmentation—5-Things-Women-Should-Know&id=2023728>.
12. Breast Implants and the FDAR page updated June 2008 reviewed by Michael Olding, MD, FACS Consumer guide to plastic surgery
13. Saline Versus Silicone Breast Implants Reviewed by Michael Olding, MD, FACS Cosmetic Plastic Surgery Costs By Denise Mann Sources: American Society for Aesthetic Plastic Surgery website. Cost: Surgeon Fees per Procedure. [page updated January 2009]
14. Anesthesia and Plastic Surger Reviewed by Ronald E. Iverson, MD, FACS
15. Ronald E. Iverson, MD, FACS, is a board-certified plastic surgeon, a member and former president of the American Society of Plastic Surgeons, a member of the American Society for Aesthetic Plastic Surgery, and an American Medical Association delegate. Dr. Iverson received his medical degree from the University of California, Los Angeles, and performed his residency at Stanford University Medical Center, General Surgery and Plastic and Reconstructive Surgery. [page updated June 2008] consumer guide to plastic surgery
16. Joe, Sky "The Addiction Of Cosmetic Surgery For Women." The Addiction Of Cosmetic Surgery For Women. 6 Mar. 2007. EzineArticles.com. 6 Jun 2009 <http://ezinearticles.com/?The-Addiction-Of-Cosmetic-Surgery-For-Women&id=463648>.

Chapter 30 Alternative Medicine

1. http://www.medic8.com/ Do Complementary and Alternative Medicine Therapies Help Menopausal Symptoms?
2. Holisticonline.comAlternative Medicine for Menopause Copyright © 2000-2002, ICBS, Inc.
3. WWW.WEMD.Com Menopause and Alternative Therapy,JUNE 8 2009
4. Alternative therapies for type 2 diabetes - Review: type 2 diabetes Alternative Medicine Review , Feb, 2002 by Lucy Dey, Anoja S. Attele, Chun-Su Yuan Health Care Industry
5. Ayurvedic Interventions for Diabetes Mellitus: A Systematic Review. Summary, Evidence Report/Technology Assessment: Number 41. AHRQ Publication No. 01-E039, June 2001. Agency for Healthcare Research and Quality, Rockville, MD. http://www.ahrq.gov/clinic/epcsums/ayurvsum.htm Search   CAM and Diabetes: A Focus on Dietary Supplements NCCAM Publication No. D416, June 2008
6. Health Care Industry Industry: Email Alert RSS Feed Alternative therapies for type 2 diabetes - Review: type 2 diabetes Alternative Medicine Review , Feb, 2002 by Lucy Dey, Anoja S. Attele, Chun-Su Yuan Complementary/Alternative Medicine (CAM) Therapies for Cholesterol Reduction The Cleveland Clinic Foundation. Chinese Herbs for Uterine Fibroids Leiomyomas of the Uterus Reduced Without Invasive Medical Procedures © Dawn M. Smith Apr 3, 2008 suite101.de
7. Alternative Medicines for Uterine Fibroids by the Editors of Consumer Guide. Chinese Herbal Medicine for Dysfunctional Uterine Bleeding: a Meta-analysis Xiang Tu, Gaomin Huang and Shengkui Tan College of Clinical Medicine, Chengdu University of Traditional Chinese Medicine, Chengdu 610075, Sichuan Province, China Meditation Health Conditions That Are Benefited By Meditation holistichealthonline.com